From Deep Within: Poetry Workshops in Nursing Homes

From Deep Within: Poetry Workshops in Nursing Homes

Carol F. Peck

The Haworth Press
New York • London

From Deep Within: Poetry Workshops in Nursing Homes has also been published as *Activities, Adaptation & Aging,* Volume 13, Number 3 1989.

The Haworth Press, Inc., 10 Alice Street, Binghamton, NY 13904-1580
EUROSPAN/Haworth, 3 Henrietta Street, London, WC2E 8LU England

Library of Congress Cataloging-in-Publication Data

Peck, Carol F.
    From deep within : poetry workshops in nursing homes / Carol F. Peck.
      p.   cm.
    "Has also been published as Activities, adaptation & aging, volume 13, number 3, 1989"–
T.p. verso.
    Bibliography: p.
    ISBN: 1-56024-622-7
    1. Poetry–Study and teaching. 2. Poetry–Authorship. 3. Poetry–Therapeutic use. 4. Aged–
Recreation. I. Title.
PN1101.P43 1989
808.1'07'152-dc19   89-30946
                                                      CIP

To Helen Anderson's blazingly accurate images and metaphors,
To Alice Balliet's apt turns of phrase and good humor,
To Joan Brindley's ready wit in every poem,
To Alice Caton's and Eleanor O'Brien's sharing of vivid
        memories of their large, loving family,
To Catherine Curtin's courage in using poetry to triumph over
        aphasia,
To Dorothy Emerson's "still small voice" centering her poems,
To Alice Kennedy's true ear for the sounds of language,
To Dorothy Yates' philosophical approach to each writing idea
        and knack for building each poem to a good last line,
To the memory of Anna Goldschmidt's zest for trying new ideas,
To the memory of Vida Hickerson's bright spirit and articulate
        descriptions,
And to the spirit of adventure of everyone who has participated in
        our group.

From Deep Within: Poetry Workshops in Nursing Homes

CONTENTS

ABOUT THE AUTHOR

Carol F. Peck, MA, has been teaching creative writing at the University of Maryland since 1971. Since 1978 she has been Writer-in-Residence at Sidwell Friends Lower School, Washington, DC, where she teaches creative writing and writes original operettas for the students to perform. As a volunteer she has led a weekly poetry workshop at the Bethesda Retirement and Nursing Center for the last 10 years. Among her poetry awards is an Avery Hopwood Award from the University of Michigan. She has published poems and articles in a number of scholarly journals and has published several songs.

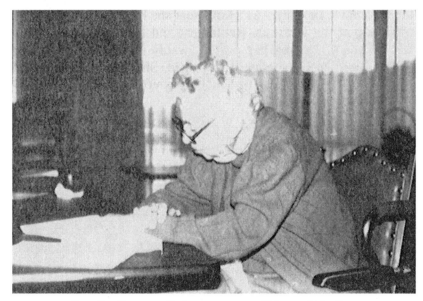
Dorothy Emerson finds many poems "deep within."
Photo by Wendy C. Webster.

What should a poem be or do?
It was a long time
Before I came to our poetry class.
I thought a poem had to rhyme;
I didn't know it would "come"
If I got myself out of the way
And just "listened."
A poem has its own message,
It already exists.
It has a message for me—
It comes from a world of ideas
That opens new thoughts and sounds.
It may not mean anything to you,
But I am learning to "be" in a new world
Now and then.
I cannot teach you how to write a poem—
Just try going "blank"
And see what comes to you from deep within.

—Dorothy Emerson, BRNC

Preface

Several writers, such as Kenneth Koch and Marc Kaminsky, have described their experiences working with older adults. But I particularly admire *Writers Have No Age: Creative Writing With Older Adults*, by Lenore M. Coberly, Jeri McCormick and Karen Updike who describe their workshops in detail, give specific lesson plans, and include a wealth of student work, as well as valuable lists of resources. It was their chapter on classes in a nursing home that encouraged me to write about my ten years of leading a weekly poetry writing group in a nursing home and to address situations that come up in a long-term workshop. For example: how do you keep thinking up new writing ideas for basically the same people every week for several years? How do you keep a project easy enough for the hesitant first-timer who keeps protesting, "I just don't think I'm any good at poetry" yet challenging enough for the skilled, experienced, sophisticated workshop veteran? These are some of the challenges, among the many joys I have faced, and quite simply I would like to share my solutions, as well as writing ideas and examples, with those who may be doing similar work. I strongly urge anyone using this book to consider it a companion to *Writers Have No Age*.

I would like to thank Jeanette Levin and Marian Dowling of Sidwell Friends School for their writing ideas, "These I Have Loved" and "Gloomy February, Magic Me!" respectively; David Anstaett of Kansas City, Missouri, for "Colors of Time of Day"; Earl Oremus of Boston's Center for Applied Special Technology for "Senses of Feeling"; and Masha Spiegel of the Charles E. Smith Jewish Day School for "What We've Known."

I am grateful to Beckie Karras for asking me in 1978 to lead this group, to the Activities Staff for their continued support, and to the many staff members at the Bethesda Retirement and Nursing Center who have helped me in many ways. And I am indebted to the members of the group and their heirs, as well as to my students at Sidwell Friends School, Washington, D.C., who generously permitted me to print their poems.

Chapter 1

Beginnings

. . . our memories are just like those of active people about us.

—Eleanor O'Brien, BRNC

MY RESPONSIBILITIES

It seemed straightforward and easy enough—as volunteer Writing Group Leader in a nursing home for one hour weekly, my duties would be to:

1. Lead a small group of interested residents in learning to write prose or poetry, as a means of self-expression and ventilation of feelings.
2. Write down a resident's thoughts if resident is unable to physically write.
3. Provide good examples of writing.
4. Encourage any gestures of self-expression.

I had been doing poetry workshops with schoolchildren (K-12), teachers, and adult college students for over 7 years, but I had no idea how these older students would compare with all my others. Should I proceed as with my college class, giving an assignment to be written during the week and brought to class to be discussed? Or should these students write in class, the way the schoolchildren did? Instinct told me the latter was better, at least to start, especially since I had no knowledge of the group's capabilities—some people might need on-the-spot encouragement and some might need to dictate their work. I could always offer "homework" to those who wished it.

WHO CAME?

The Activities Staff did an excellent job of assembling my first class through personal invitations to residents they thought would be most interested in a poetry workshop. Those who responded were well educated and, for the most part, well read; a few had even published some poetry or prose. Of the twelve or fourteen who came that first day, about ten came back week after week, forming a core group for most of that first year. However, the turnout each week was unpredictable — with a few drop-outs and drop-ins likely — and sometimes illness caused absences. Over the years the core group has changed, of course, with only one of the original members still in it, but always there has been this solid center with fluid edges, and many of the current members have been with me for many years. We have had a few men join the class, from time to time, but most of the poets have been women.

WHERE AND HOW DID WE WORK?

For the first session, and every session since then, the Activities Staff brought the wheelchair-bound to an area of the Craft Room, which has turned out to be an excellent location: it is a quiet room big enough to hold both a movable bed and a table that accommodates about twelve chairs and wheelchairs. They also have several individual folding tables in case of overflow. There is an easel with a huge table of white "chart" paper on it and a thick black marker so I can write notes or guidelines for the class. This tablet is much easier to see than a blackboard.

Just as I had sensed that we should write in class, each time, I also knew that because of the unpredictability of the group, each week, I could not really run this like a course in which activities build on — depend on — previous activities; I had to present a new, self-contained writing idea, each meeting, one which could be completed in twenty to thirty minutes — one of the main reasons for sticking to poetry rather than short story or essay.

GETTING STARTED: PRIMING THE PUMP

Looking at these friendly and expectant faces I realized that these people had finished school before I was even born, and no doubt many had some ideas about poetry very different from mine. So I told them that I was a poet who especially enjoyed helping students of all ages to write and that even if they had always thought of poetry as rhymed, metered lines such as they had read and memorized in school, I wanted to show them ways in which they could use language to bring ideas and feelings alive on paper, to connect with their poetic selves. They would not have to worry about following strict patterns or rules but could open up their imaginations and surprise themselves.

Because I knew that I had to provide enough focus and structure that the novices, the hesitant writers would feel secure, yet enough freedom that the more experienced would not feel restricted or that I was telling them what to write, I started this group the way I nearly always start any group—with the concept of IMAGE, of making pictures with words. Vivid specifics that *show* rather than *tell* are the backbone of much good writing, both prose as well as poetry, I said, and we would start with a group effort to warm up our mental image-makers. I had prepared the pattern for what children often call a "wheel poem" or "sun poem": I covered a large piece of cardboard (24" × 30") with white sign paper from an art store, and using colored markers I drew around a luncheon plate in the middle and then made straight lines radiating like spokes from the edge of the circle to the edges of the board, about 20 total. I told them I would write a generalization, a "big idea" in the circle, and they would create images, "word pictures" to bring it alive, which I would write on the lines. I wrote "Blue is . . ." in the center and then, some quickly, some hesitantly, they supplied images like "the look of twilight," "a border of flowers," "my daughter's eyes." Next I asked them to use all five senses to make images for the sounds, smells, tastes, and textures of blue—and that led to "the crash of ocean waves," "the heavenly aroma of fresh blueberry pie," "the cool taste of sherbet," "the soft warmth of a baby's blanket," etc. By the time we had filled the lines, they were really warming up to the idea and openly appreciative of each other's contributions—essential for the success of a group effort. Best of all, they had more ideas than we had lines for, so it was time for individual writing.

STIMULATING WITHOUT SUFFOCATING

I told them that they could use this sensory image technique to build color poems of their own, but I first read them several widely varying examples: two from Mary O'Neill's *Hailstones and Halibut Bones*, whose rhymes pleased them; William Carlos Williams' un-rhymed "Primrose" (not in the Bibliography), in which he repeats the name of the color, says it is *not* a color, and proceeds with a series of far-reaching images to show what it *is*; and a few short, unrhymed color poems by elementary schoolchildren which had wonderfully fresh images:

GREY

Grey is mysterious, like morning haze;
Grey is soft and bumpy
   but feels like touching the softest breeze
  that only the most patient and calmest person can feel;
It tastes like warm cocoa in the early morning,
Like a branch falling, breaking a total silence;
Grey sounds like a rug sliding across the smoothest floor,
Or like the Indian chief whispering commands to his braves.

—Patrick DeLeon, Grade 3

BLACK

Black is like the darkness in a faraway cave;
Black tastes like black licorice;
Black sounds like a wolf calling in the night under a full moon;
Black smells like smoke;
Black feels cold and stiff.

—Ben Smith, Grade 1

I think it is important to read several examples whenever possi-ble—all students want to know what *you* have in mind regarding the assignment—and to present a wide variety of approaches, so that just about anything a participant writes will be within scope; they are bound to respond in different ways, and you want to stress that there are no right or wrong answers—just pleasure in writing down ideas. On the big white tablet I summarized the assignment: "(1) Choose a color you feel strongly about—love or hate. (2) Bring it alive through *sensory images*—describe how it looks, sounds, smells, tastes, feels, and makes you feel inside—not necessarily in that order. Try to *show* your feeling about it without stating it."

TAKING DICTATION

A few members of the group could not write for themselves, because of paralyzed limbs, so I offered to write for them. I had never taken dictation from adults, but I just proceeded conversationally: "What color would you like to write about?" Because of the guidelines I had already mentioned to the group and the examples I had read, the dictators clearly understood what we were doing, and all I had to do was occasional reminding—"You have mentioned its look and sound, but what about its texture?"

A RICHNESS OF POEMS

When our hour was up, everyone had written something, even the lady who had announced, very firmly, that she was just there to sit on the sidelines and listen. I had cajoled her into letting me at least push her wheelchair up to the table and put paper and pencil in front of her—"I know you just want to listen, but this way, if an idea happens to come along, you will be ready for it." After collecting all the work, I read it aloud, because some had trouble seeing what they had just written and I wanted to make sure I understood everything prior to typing it up. The writing ranged from lists of things of a particular color that the writer liked, to real poems bringing the color alive, to poems using color as just a departure—for example, blue reminded one lady of her cats' eyes, so she wrote about how much she loved her blue-eyed cats. *All* results were valid, I stressed—that is the beauty of poetry.

WHAT THEY WROTE

YELLOW

I choose my favorite color, yellow —
Yellow is a cheerful color;
Yellow is car lights on a foggy day;
Yellow is a maple tree in the fall,
A lemon lying in the dish and waiting
To make your mouth pucker;
Yellow is all around us
In the moon,
In the tomato waiting to turn bright red;
Yellow looks and tastes just like a banana.

—Joan Brindley, BRNC

RED

Red is the color of the setting sun;
It smells of the night approaching;
It says to us, "Go to sleep."
Red is the color of corals that grow in the water —
They want to adorn a child's neck;
They go to sleep when taken out of the water,
But they stay red forever;
They smell of the water they left;
They would like to be back in there,
Getting alive again.
Red is the color of the most beautiful rose,
Smelling very nice, fading only when the rose dies.
Red is what I like best in a dress,
It reflects one's cheek;
It makes one look young and pretty;
It says, "Please wear me a lot —
You will look nice when you do."

—Anna Goldschmidt, BRNC

BROWN

Brown is nature's stabilizer;
It's the color of the earth from which all else rises,
The warm, moist retainer of the elements;
Brown is stretching limbed trees
   holding tight to leaves that try ever to rise;
Brown is black coffee, hot chocolate and old sherry;
It's the color of a struggling race,
The clinging warmth of fur and Brahms,
And the color of mood most deeply in thought.

                                   —*Helen L. Anderson, BRNC*

RED

Red, Red, Red, Red,
It is not a color,
It is the fire in a hearth
On a gloomy, rainy day;
It is the final glow of sunset;
It is the sun itself high in the sky;
It is the sudden flash of a cardinal
Darting through the trees;
It is a sumac bush in the fall,
Putting forth its last burst of beauty
Before the sleep of winter;
Energy, Energy, Energy, Energy!

                                     —*Dorothy Yates, BRNC*

GOLD

The gold of the sunset
Enfolds my heart,
Binding it in love's glory.

                                     —*Leila King, BRNC*

FOLLOWUP TO WRITING

As I had promised, I took their handwritten work home, typed it up in capital letters onto a ditto master, and duplicated copies for everyone in the workshop. The Activities Department reimbursed me for ditto masters and paper, and I was able to use the machine I used for schoolwork. Over the ten years, I have used all capitals on a regular typewriter (okay), a primary typewriter (better), and finally, a Macintosh computer using the New York 18 font which is the same size as the primary typewriter's. The printout is photocopied by the nursing home right before each session (best). The

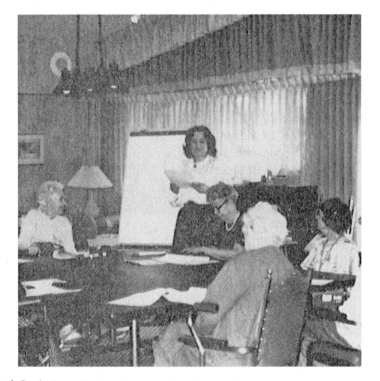

Carol Peck (standing) enjoys reading the previous week's poems along with (l. to r.) Eleanor O'Brien, Catherine Curtin, Dorothy Emerson and Dona Clapp.
Photo by Wendy C. Webster.

participants never complained, but the black photocopies are clearly easier for them to read than the purple dittos.

The only editing I did, or have ever done, was to correct spelling and occasionally to arrange a paragraph as lines of poetry, when that format seemed to strengthen the writing—I tried to let the rhythm of the writing determine that. At our next meeting, they were thrilled to see their work "in print," and we started the session with each poet reading his or her work aloud. Having copies of the poems in front of them was a special help to those who were hard of hearing. I made a brief comment on each piece, saying what I liked best about it—the vividness of an image, the sound of a phrase, the saving of the best line for last, etc. Over the years I have found that students of all ages learn more from what you build up than from what you tear down, in their writing, and will strive to do what you praise in their and others' work.

I have never done much with revision, in this workshop; our time and often their energies are limited, and they seem more interested in trying the new idea than in fiddling with last week's. Of course there have been a few poets who have wanted to revise and refine, but I have helped them in individual conferences.

> The reason I like to write poetry is
> I can express my thoughts
> Without disturbing anyone.
>
> —*Pauline Immerman, BRNC*

Chapter 2

Special Challenges

We were off to a good start and continued to follow that structure of first reading and admiring last week's poems and then tackling a new writing idea. As the weeks, months and years rolled by, however, things came up that I had not anticipated and had to learn to deal with.

UNPREDICTABLE CLASS SIZE

Being accustomed to stable classes whose numbers varied little from week to week, I found it a bit unsettling, at first, never to know if there would be four or fourteen and how many would be newcomers. Gradually I became used to it, especially as I got to know the "core group" better and felt more like their friend than "teacher." The self-containment of each session helped—had the participants been taking homework assignments back to their rooms and perhaps missing the next week or returning empty-handed, they would not have had a sense of accomplishment, there would not have been the poems to read aloud and discuss, and newcomers would have had a hard time understanding what we were all about. I learned to urge them to finish their poems in class, if humanly possible, as unfinished work taken away with them often got lost or forgotten by the time we met again. And many have told me that they feel more inspired to write when they are part of a group all working on the same project. Indeed, the few times we had to have individuals write in their rooms, because of an influenza quarantine, it just did not work as well—and they were the first to realize and comment on that.

I also learned to take a few minutes to explain very briefly to newcomers, *before* they protested, as a few did, "This isn't *poetry* — it doesn't even rhyme! I never saw poetry like *this*!" that we were a poetry workshop because we were exploring our feelings and experiences in writing — that we did not necessarily follow traditional forms, and that sometimes we wrote in prose paragraphs.

INSECURITIES

Occasionally people would join the group who were very unsure of themselves and kept saying things like, "I really shouldn't be here — I was never good at poetry." Or, "I don't know why I am here — I am not prepared — I didn't have time to work on anything." They were worried that it would be like school with hard assignments and right or wrong answers. Sometimes reading the poems from the previous session alleviated their fears, but often I had to reassure them over and over that there was no right or wrong and that they could do it, too. I never forced anyone to write, but I did ask them to sit at the table with pencil and paper in front of them — just to be ready. After the others had been writing for several minutes, I would confer with the insecure member; if he or she had written anything at all down, I would read it and say something like, "Oh, you have a *good* start," — point to an image I liked and say so, and then encourage, "Keep going!" The writer would say, "Is it really okay?" And I would say, "Yes — I like what you are doing with it." If there was nothing on the paper yet, I would ask what he or she was thinking about the subject and say, "Yes — good ideas — why don't you write them down?" Usually that was all it took for someone to become comfortable with our poetry writing, but a few needed that kind of bolstering and coaching every single time, and it became a ritual.

DISRUPTERS

I had worried about what I would do if someone joined the group who was too confused or disruptive to participate, but the few times that happened, either I was able to quiet a "talker" by saying, very low, right into the person's ear, "It's our quiet writing time, now" or else an Activities Staff member appeared and skillfully, gently steered him or her to another activity. Staff members were always nearby in their office — that is essential, I think, in case of a medical or other emergency.

NONTALKERS

A tougher problem was the occasional person from whom I was taking dictation but who seemed to have nothing to say. Generally I first went through the guidelines, the "leading questions" I had written up on the big tablet, which got most people started, but once in a while I had to start from scratch: for example, "What were you thinking about when I was talking about snow?" or "Do you like to see it snow? Why?" Or I might think back to a more successful interview and say, "You once told me about your job with the government — all those people you supervised downtown — were there ever 'snow days' then?" If you can connect your personality with the other person's, you can start to communicate, and that leads to his or her sharing thoughts you can write down.

SPEECH DIFFICULTIES

Occasionally I have had to take dictation from people whose speech has been impaired by stroke; they know they are hard to understand but can become frustrated if unable to communicate at all. When I could understand some of the words, I used those as my guide — starting with the known to question my way into the unknown, letting non-verbal signals, such as nods or head-shaking, guide me. When I could not understand, again I started with what I knew they had heard me read and what they could read on the tablet, talking in a way that they could respond to non-verbally: "There are a lot of textures — would you say that red is rough? . . . smooth? . . . prickly? . . . slimy?" . . . etc. It was not as hard as it sounds — I soon learned the personalities of these people and grew in my understanding of their speech and ideas.

VEERING FROM THE TOPIC

At first I wondered what to do when somebody wrote a poem about something totally different from the idea of the day, but I learned that that was not important — what was important was that he or she was writing about something worth sharing. In the readings I simply said, "Mr. or Mrs. _____ has written about _____." One lady spent several sessions writing two to four lines of Joyce Kilmer's "Trees," presenting it as something she had been working on for some time; when I typed these pieces up, I simple wrote, "Contributed by _____." At the readings I thanked her for remembering and sharing lines from a poem that many people like. As it turned out, she seldom remembered our sessions from one week to the next but thoroughly enjoyed each one and occasionally wrote extremely good original poems . . . and one day, in the nursing home library, I found a volume of her poems published many years ago.

FRAIL POPULATION

Because I was used to teaching energetic young children, restless high school students, and driving, motivated adult college students, I was not prepared for the limited stamina of the nursing home poets. For the most part they were very bright, alert, and well educated, and it was hard to realize that they could not — metaphorically — juggle several balls at a time. However, I learned to tune into their pace, while I was there, to give sufficient guidelines for them to write without a tiring "overkill" of examples, to sit rather than bounce around, to write along with them occasionally, if nobody needed me to take dictation, and not to be surprised by their occasional dozing off. Just beyond the French doors of our room is a beautiful garden, and I have come to love really looking at it. There are also some cats who have grown up in that room, and I, a non-cat person, have grown to enjoy them. In short I have learned to slow down, to appreciate, to live for the moment, to guard against rushing these writers — and they are the ones who have taught me.

CHALLENGING THE PROS WITHOUT SCARING OFF NEWCOMERS

Over the ten years, however, the biggest challenge has been coming up with writing ideas that would stimulate the experienced "core group" without scaring off any newcomers. The best solutions I have found are:

1. Present *specific* ideas — rather than "Let's write poems about summer," say, "Let's write poems *to* summer — welcoming it, describing how it looks, sounds, tastes, feels, and smells, how it makes *us* feel, asking it questions, perhaps, and telling it what we *don't* like about it."

2. Do group brainstorming, perhaps — write down on the big tablet their answers to such questions as "What does the word 'summer' make you think of? What are summer's sounds, smells, tastes?" etc.

3. Offer examples of several different approaches, ideally a mixture of a few professional poems from more than one century and some by students of varying ages, a mixture not always possible, of course. For example, "Sumer Is Icumen In," Isabelle Gardner's "Summer Remembered" (not in any anthology in the Bibliography but worth hunting down) or Christina Rossetti's "Summer," a nursing home resident's poem or two, and a current third grader's comparison of summer to a playful puppy. (*Note:* Because I do workshops with schoolchildren, I have access to a wealth of young writers' work; however, the Bibliography lists several volumes containing poems by children.)

SUMMER

The buzz of bees
Working busily in the clover,
The brilliant color of birds
Flashing past our eye,
The fragrance of sun on pine needles,
Softening the sound of tiny footsteps;
The cool flavor of pure spring water
Refreshes the traveller

On his lazy wanderings
Through the restful days of summer.

—Dorothy Yates, BRNC

SUMMER REMEMBERED

Playing games after dinner
When it was getting dark
And you started to see alligators;
You smelled the grass
And you could hear happy sounds
Of children laughing and playing.
And after the games
It felt great to be in bed,
Thinking about what you had done
During the day;
The sheets felt cool and smooth;
You dreamed of happiness and gaiety.

—Betty Graham, BRNC

SUMMER IS A PUPPY

Summer is a puppy;
It's not there until you
Least expect it . . .
Then it pops out of nowhere
And flops on you;
Summer sits and watches you
And is quiet for a time;
Then, as fast as it can,
It runs toward you and tickles you
And licks you so much that
You scream and laugh;
Then it rolls in the grass,
And if you play too rough,
It bites.
Summer runs around the earth
Spreading sunshine;
It comes to one place and blazes . . .

But then it runs off
And winter comes . . .
And I'm sad.

—Marc Iannucci, Grade 4

Once in a while a member of the group has requested that I tell them a week in advance what the next writing idea will be, but most have said that they wanted to be surprised; I try to strike a happy medium—occasionally giving advance notice for an idea that I think will benefit from prior reflection but, for the most part, surprising them. Besides, I do not always *know* a week in advance what I'll be doing!

The remainder of this book is devoted to a selection of ideas I have used successfully over the past ten years, complete with guidelines and examples that can be used to inspire other nursing home writing groups. Not all of them blaze new trails—many repeat what all of us who teach creative writing have recommended all along, such as reliance on sensory imagery, vivid language, compression, etc. The ideas are organized into six sections: three of them deal with poetic techniques, and the other three are more subject-oriented. For each idea I have listed "guidelines," or "leading questions," occasionally suggested some variations of the project, which help keep the core group challenged when we repeat an assignment, and given several example poems, including several from the group. Whenever possible, I have cited professional poems that would be good examples, as some group members love hearing poems they read—even memorized—in school; others enjoy hearing what contemporary poets are doing; and all of them respond to each other's work and to children's writing—children have such a fresh view of the world that they are natural poets, and their poems never fail to delight my class in the nursing home. When selecting the examples by the children and by the nursing home class, I have tried to show the wide range of their responses.

All books mentioned are listed in the Bibliography, and all professional poems cited, unless noted otherwise, appear in one or more of the anthologies listed in the Bibliography.

Chapter 3

Writing Projects

POETRY

Sometimes you feel you're foolish to do it,
But then you realize that you're foolish
If you don't!

—Leila King, BRNC

A. COME TO YOUR SENSES

Poems calling for sensory imagery make excellent writing projects for beginner and experienced poet alike and are especially good for starting a writing group; our five senses are readily available to us and help us show our ideas and feelings in a way that others can experience directly. I stressed vivid images early on, hoping that people would get in the habit of using them in all their work.

After several sessions, when the group seemed quite comfortable with the writing projects we were doing, I introduced the idea of unity, variety and progression necessary for any good work of art — unity is the theme that makes the poem hang together; variety is the use of many different images to give the poem energy; progression is the arrangement of images or ideas in a good dramatic order with the best one coming last. From time to time, after that, I would remind them to seek variety and to build a good progression; the writing idea provided the unity.

1. Color Revisited

People respond to color so readily that periodically I have repeated that first writing idea about five times over the last ten years — at first I worried about repetition, but those who had written color poems before never seemed to mind, and each time I tried to have new examples so it would not seem like a stale rerun. A good stimulator is to scatter on the table several sheets of every color of 9" × 12" construction paper you can find. You could use brightly colored objects, as well — ribbons, fabrics, toys, blocks, flowers, etc. As all writing teachers know, hands-on stimuli are especially effective. You could also try a variation.

(a) Colors of Times of Day

For this poem the writer links various times of day to different colors and shows *why* he or she feels that way.
Guidelines:

- List all the times of day the group can name — including such lovely names as "dusk," "twilight," "dawn," etc.
- List as many colors as possible, including shades, blends, and descriptive names like "flamingo pink," "lime green," and "chocolate brown."
- Summarize the writing idea: "Describe the color of at least three times of day — be sure to show *why* each is that color to you."

Examples:

Morning is blue
like the early morning sky
because I am fresh and
ready for a new day.
At noon I feel light green
like new grass in spring
because I am so full of ideas.
In the afternoon I feel yellow
like the sun at its brightest point
because I am at my brightest point.

In the evening I feel pink
like the sunset
because I am happy.
And late at night I feel black
because I am thinking of a new day.

—Laura Graham, Grade 3

In the morning it is light yellow from
    the sun just coming out;
At noon it is hungry red like lunchtime
    and hot;
In afternoon it is blue and boring;
Evening is sparkling white
    after you have taken a bath;
Night is black and silver
    from the night and stars.

—Nikki Huvelle, Grade 2

Morning is a new, fresh white, pink and yellow—
It starts another day and
All the rest goes down from there,
As far as I am concerned;
At noon the colors darken
And visibility becomes more difficult to me;
Some afternoons have a surprise in them,
Like a visitor—red popping up;
Evening and night are a nice, comfortable warm gray,
    where you can seek refuge from surprise.

—Dorothy Skinker, BRNC

Morning is yellow like the sun—it makes me happy;
Noontime is misty gray—it makes me feel depressed;
Afternoon, the gray just gets thicker and darker,
And as it gets darker at night,
I get more depressed;
The darkness is what gets to you and makes you
Look forward to the next morning.

—Margaret Hayes, BRNC

Morning is a glowing color, pinkish red, an inspirational color, summoning me to make the most of the dawning day. I like morning because I enjoy making a list of things I hope to do that day.

Noontime is yellow, the apogee of the day, the time when I check off all the tasks I have accomplished in the morning and scan those remaining for afternoon. It is a respite, a time for a brief relaxation in the brilliant yellow of noon before beginning the afternoon.

Afternoon is orange as the yellow passes; and then comes the serene green which is so pleasant as an end to a full day, a beautiful day beginning with a rosy "Salutation to the Dawn."

Night is brown to black, offering surcease from toil and, I always hope, a lovely feeling of accomplishment. Night brings sleep, which is entered by a song in my mind of thankfulness and a return to the color green as I recapture scenes of green meadows, pale yellow moonlight, and silvery still waters.

—Vida Hickerson, BRNC

Morning is a bugle that wakes you up—
It is the color of different kinds of horses;
Tom Payton and I broke horses for the Army Remount Service;
Afternoon and evening are different colors,
But I am color blind and cannot see them
Unless they have designs on them.

—John Mann, BRNC

(b) Noisiest Color

This idea focuses on one color and one sense; since they will be writing about noise, it helps to have the group collect some "noisy words" first—many will remember having learned about onomatopoeia in school.

Guidelines:

—After telling the group the idea, spend a few minutes asking
   for "noisy words" which you write down on the tablet—
   "bang," "crash," "boom," "shriek," "clang," etc.
—Remind them: "Be sure to use a variety of specifics to 'prove'
   that the color is the noisiest. Put your strongest image at the
   end."

Examples:

The noisiest color is purple—
You can't keep it quiet
No matter what you try!
It wants to be heard.
It sounds like bells ringing—
It says, "Here I am—look at me!"
It makes a lot of noise when you look at it—
Just don't expect it to be quiet!

—Dorothy Oest, BRNC

THE NOISIEST COLORS

Clang, shriek, shout, scream, bang, clash,
Crash, boom, blast, cling, ring, burst—
Orange is a very noisy color, maybe the noisiest of all—
It shrieks at you, it crashes out of a bunch of zinnias,
It clashes with yellow or gold,
It bursts out of the tree when oranges there are ripe,
It sings, "My juice is the healthiest you can find";
It booms when you have a dish of fruit, calling, "Pick me out!"
Black is the noisiest color of all—
Death wears a black dress,
Black berries cling to the tree, saying,
"Don't eat me, I am poisonous!"

—Anna Goldschmidt, BRNC

The noisiest color is blue—
Navy uniform,
The sheik, his tent, his cape,

Thunder,
Cannon at Fort Myer in the morning at 6:00,
Clappin' for the Pope,
A blue car in a crash!
Blue fireworks open with a bang and give you a thrill.
Opera stars burst when they sing the blues!
Bridesmaids in blue walk to the organ blasting
"Here Comes the Bride!"

— Gertrude Robinson, BRNC

2. Celebrating Single Senses

Have students write a poem celebrating just one sense — favorite sights, sounds, smells, tastes, or textures. I found it worked well to have the whole class working on the same sense at the same time, knowing that next week they would all write about another. Some years I gave it an additional focus such as "Celebrating Light," "Tiny Sounds," or "Silences in Life," and one year the spring was so glorious that we devoted four weeks to it: "Looks of Spring," "Sounds of Spring," "Smells and Tastes of Spring," and "Textures of Spring." This could be done with other seasons, of course, or with a day of the week, holiday, etc., seeing how much variety one can achieve when limited to one sense. (*NOTE*: In *Writers Have No Age*, pp. 99-100, there is an excellent list of professional poems concentrating on various senses.)

Guidelines:

- Ask students for examples of favorite *outdoor* sights (or sounds, smells, etc.) and write them on the large tablet; ask for some *indoor* ones, some throughout the day, some from *childhood* and, for contrast, some they do *not* like.
- Summarize in writing: "Write a poem celebrating the sense of sight, perhaps focusing on a particular season or time of your life. Choose a wide variety of specifics and put them into their best order."

Examples:

FEASTS FOR THE EYES

I like to look at chocolate — the brown color;
I like to look at chicken, after it is cooked;
I like to look at mountains — so different from anything you see,
   several colors of green and blue and also reddish;
I like to watch the waves at the ocean,
   coming up and going back —
   everything is blue and green and white sand;
I like to look at buildings in Washington —
   especially the White House and its furnishings;
I like to see the rain — you feel you don't have to get up
   but can just stay in bed!

— Vanetta Bealle, BRNC

CELEBRATING LIGHT

We celebrate light:
The sun — how it glistens in the sky,
   how it dances on waves,
   how it brings life to the world;
Moonlight — glowing in the black of night,
   shimmering softly on a lake and
   making us feel peaceful;
Flashes of mystery from a lighthouse that makes
   a portrait of itself on the ocean;
The mystery of imagination,
The sparkling joy of knowledge,
The glow of friendship. . . .

— From a composite poem by a group of 4th graders

I celebrate light:
The reflection of a sinking sun on the clouds;
The strange shadowy things I saw at the bottom of the sea —
   they told me it came from phosphorescence;
They were right — that's the reason I can see my watch in the
   dark;
So many sources of light —

But all the candles in the world and
All the fires laid in the fireplaces
Aren't much good without matches!

—Joan Brindley, BRNC

I CELEBRATE LIGHT

From the first glimmer of light at dawn
Through the bright heat of noon
To the waning glow of twilight
And the sharp stabs of starlight
To the final soft blanket of moonlight
Our days and nights are punctured by light;
So our minds are pierced by thoughts
Brought into light by knowledge,
    experience and companionship.

—Dorothy Yates, BRNC

NOTE: When we write about sounds, I spend a few minutes writing down examples of onomatopoeia, as in the "Noisiest Color" assignment, and encourage the writers to use them to enhance their poems.

CELEBRATE SOUND

Sounds are the keys that open the
Hoarding boxes of time stored
    and tightly packed memories,
And how suddenly they are released
    with the remembrances
When one hears the lock of an oar on a rowboat,
The far-off plea of a train whistle late at night,
The screech of a bat cruelly cornered against
    the dining room ceiling,
The soft brushy sounds of someone coming home
    late at night,
And the loveliness of family noises
    getting ready to eat;

How quickly pushed aside these brief thoughts
And locked away from the noise of now
To be re-opened at another time by
The loudness of memories kept.

—Helen L. Anderson, BRNC

SOUNDS

The large parking lot where I parked my car at work was surrounded by uncut bushes and shrubs and therefore an inviting refuge for small animals and birds. At the entrance you were always greeted by a bobwhite's call. It pleased me, as I had never heard the call before, but it was so distinct that there could be no doubt. It was not a robin, and each person knew, because he would repeat and repeat.

I love the sound of all music. It does something for your soul and for your body, too. It was the sound of music that rescued me from the black night inside me after surgery. One nurse noticed my foot moving to the sound of music, and another nurse brought me conscious and alert when she directed, "Now, when I say 'doo-dah,' you say 'do-dah.'" Then she would point her finger at me and say, "Now, you say 'doo-dah,'" and we wound sing the rest of the song together, as it is an old, familiar song.

—Eleanor O'Brien, BRNC

TINY SOUNDS

The tiniest sounds are . . .
A caterpillar crawling,
Parked cars,
Clouds floating,
Somebody closing a door softly,
Somebody going to a zoo,
A giraffe eating,
A tree looking at the sky.

—Jonathan Murphy, Pre-Kindergarten

The tiniest sounds are . . .
Bees buzzing,

Butterflies moving their wings,
People clapping softly,
Somebody having quiet time,
Flowers growing in the summer;
The sky is really quiet.

— *Sarah Bickart, Pre-Kindergarten*

The tiniest sounds come to a soul at peace,
The beat of your own heart while dreaming
Of things to do in the coming days,
The bright flame moving in a deep fireplace,
The movement of a silken cover warming
One's arms, back and legs,
The book you love while turning its page,
The wind softly sighing past,
The crickets chirping in the grass
As the eyes slowly close for the night
And all fantasies take flight.

— *Marie Huff, BRNC*

Tiny sounds are:
A fly putting his feet on the ground,
A bee chasing people,
A cat clinging among the drapes,
Worms that shake their heels over every occasion!

— *Rosalyn Fain, BRNC*

SILENCES IN LIFE

Silence — how many kinds are there?
The comfortable silence of peaceful sleep,
The held-in silence of held-in anger,
And all those between;
I had never thought of the different silences
Till now — it's overwhelming.

— *Alice Kennedy, BRNC*

I do not enjoy silences, usually —
I'd give my eyeteeth for someone to talk to;

I like silence when I read;
When my teenage grandchildren are overly silent,
They are usually up to some mischief;
They say silence is golden—perhaps it is;
A silent garden is lovely, and I enjoy it;
Silence gives one a feeling of peace of mind
And should be appreciated as such.

—Cecile Jaffe Newburg, BRNC

Having never been silent, I really don't know what it's all about, and I probably won't be silent again until Gabriel blows his horn— then I won't have much choice in the matter.

But I have experienced the tranquility of a garden, the quiet in a church, the quiet of election night when we lost and were ready to bang someone's head for not bringing in their election district!

One time I am silent is when I'm trying to think of what to write in Poetry Class!

—Alice Balliet, BRNC

SOUNDS OF SPRING

The gentle sounds of spring
Replace the roar of winter storms—
The trill of bird songs,
The buzz of insects,
The patter of spring showers,
The bleat of lambs newly arrived,
The laughter of children at outdoor play,
All life welcomes a beloved season.

—Dorothy Yates, BRNC

SOUNDS OF SPRING

Spring is a secret—she just appears;
Sometimes it's dark outdoors, yet you look again
    and see a bunch of noisy white;
Spring splashes and jumps the rope of today,
    clapping hands;
Winter is over and gone;

Now I'll write my friends the good news
Spring has whispered in my ears:
"Live the new life of today."

—Dorothy Emerson, BRNC

SOUNDS OF FALL

A squirrel scolds a bluejay
  and the bluejay screams back;
A rustle, a crackle and a snap,
  and a deer steps quietly out of a bush;
A drip, drip, drip, as drips slide off a leaf
  and drown down into a puddle after a storm;
A squirrel's tail flickers and whispers,
  "Fall is here";
A deep groan comes from a bear
  as he lumbers off to his home;
A cricket chirps and a bluejay screams in a way
  that is said, "You can only chirp";
A night wind rustles through the leaves
  and the night creatures are left with this poem.

—Jordan Press, Grade 3

CELEBRATE SMELLS

The enticing smell of freshly brewed coffee
Invites us to arise and start the day
With the promise of pleasures to come;
The blend of fragrances of Christmas cookies, cakes and candies
Brings back memories of past Christmas joys
  and the anticipation of new ones;
The crunch of newly fallen snow under our eager feet
Promises sleigh bells and happy rides in the beautiful countryside
With the clean smell of recently washed air;
The odor of burning logs in the fireplace promises a restful sleep.

—Dorothy Yates, BRNC

SMELLS

I like very much the smell of the ocean;
I like the smell of coffee;
I like the smell of flowers, but they remind me of a funeral;
I like to smell a fire in the fireplace and to sit in front of it;
I like the smell of steak;
I like to smell horses and dogs —
It reminds me of when I worked for the Cavalry;
I like the smell and sound of a cannonade — when 24 go off
    in sequence
   to salute a President;
I *don't* like to smell a pigsty or fresh manure.

—John Mann, BRNC

CELEBRATE TASTE

We read maps and translate books
To study other lands and learn how others live;
Our appetites are greedy for the gossip of geography;
But we could close our eyes, muff our ears and yet
Learn most of all from the simple art of eating
What other cultures have thriven on;
There are overheated dishes from overheated lands
And seafood from great long shores and twisted rivers,
Meats long roasted or eaten raw,
Grapes and wine from sun-sifted hills,
And cereals that have fed strength since time began,
And in each of us forever the bonded remembrance
Of our childhood foods.

—Helen L. Anderson, BRNC

TASTE

"Simple Simon met a pieman
Going to the fair,
Said Simple Simon to the pieman,
'Let me taste your ware.'"

Taste—how it rules our lives from the real tastes of heavenly chocolate mousse and bland squash, which my husband calls "tasteless insipidity," to the metaphorical use of the word as a taste for many other things, such as clothes, music, architecture, paintings.

Edward Fitzgerald called taste the feminine of genius, whatever that may mean, and a man is judged by his tastes for women, wine and Cuban cigars.

A woman's tastes, if expensive, can prove her undoing; however, a taste for beauty seems an inborn trait which refines the entire race.

But the taste that comes most often to my mind in this period of daily-released hostages is a *taste of freedom*!

—Vida Hickerson, BRNC

CELEBRATE TEXTURES

Textures—some we like—
The softness and smoothness of young skin,
The slippery slidiness of satin,
The warm bouncy feeling of hay in the hayloft
As you lie there listening to your parents calling
That it's time for supper;
Some we don't like—
The wiggly, smelly, slippery worms,
The pointed, sometimes prickly ends of a comb,
The prickly, stabbing feel of a thorn
As you try to pick that rose,
My mother's oatmeal which was full of lumps.

—Joan Brindley, BRNC

Eleanor and I had blue ratine dresses when we were little—
It was not a smooth fabric
But had little soft loops all over it;
We wore them to church—
I felt special when I wore it.

—Alice Caton, BRNC

I like velvet, smooth and like flowers —
Once I found some velvet things in a trunk,
But I don't know what they were;
Some of my family had velvet dresses.
I like the texture of flowers — they feel like velvet should;
I like satin — it makes me think of old-time dresses;
I don't like snails — I can't imagine how anybody could eat them!
I don't like sandpaper — it reminds me of cleaning off irons.

— *Vanetta Bealle, BRNC*

3. Senses of Feeling

There are many kinds of poems that are strengthened by imagery appealing to all five senses — like the color poem. One is the "feeling" poem, in which an emotion is described in terms of its color, sound, smell, taste, and texture.

Guidelines:

— List many emotions on the tablet — supplied by the group, if you wish.
— List the five senses and discuss how a feeling can be brought alive through these — add "movement" to the five senses.
— Summarize in writing: "Choose a feeling and bring it alive by describing its color, sound, smell, taste, texture, and movement — not necessarily in that order — but in the best order for your poem."

Examples:

ANGER

Anger is red, because if you get majorly mad, you could turn red;
Anger sounds like five elephants playing hopscotch on your roof;
Anger tastes like tiger-kidney pie;
Anger smells like a skunk eating a couple of rotten eggs;
Anger slithers unseen through the water and dense forests;
Anger looks like a snake, so that it can scare people away that
    notice it.

— *Webster McBride, Grade 4*

CURIOSITY

Curiosity is . . .
Gold, silver and light blue,
Very whispery;
It has no taste at all;
It smells like fresh bread from the oven;
It looks like a chewed carrot stick;
It just jumps from cupboard to cupboard;
It makes me feel like Curious George.

—Mariah Steinwinter, Grade 1

LONELINESS

Loneliness is a color nobody has invented;
Loneliness is a silent bird flying in the blue sky that never ends;
Loneliness is the sound of leaves rustling in a quiet forest;
Loneliness is a big rock in the middle of nowhere;
Loneliness sounds like the wind making the flowers dance;
Loneliness tastes very bitter;
Loneliness smells like fish in a pond;
It looks like the owl on Athena's shoulder;
It crawls;
It makes me unhappy.

—Justine Lassman, Grade 2

I choose Joy—
It sounds tinkly
And sticks to my tongue;
It looks like a mountain stream
Rippling down the mountain side
In its blue-white foam;
It makes me feel loved and belonging
And takes away the smell of Fear.

—Dorothy Emerson, BRNC

Anger is my choice of emotion —
Its color is red
And it sounds like a lion in the jungle;
Anger is very rancid and stale;
It attacks!
It is just terrible.

—*Catherine J. Curtin, BRNC*

Resentment is built as high as a Rocky Mountain
By suppressing complaints when other people
Offend or attack you;
It is black;
It sounds like the drum of rain on a tin roof;
It is tasteless because it lacks good ingredients;
It smells like someone who has been eating garlic;
It has no form, since it does not come from good feelings;
It moves like a flash of lightning.

—*Eleanor O'Brien, BRNC*

Happiness is burnt orange —
It sounds like a Beethoven violin sonata;
Happiness tastes like chocolate mousse;
It smells like Shalimar;
It glides through the air like a balloon;
It makes me feel euphoric!

—*Cecile Jaffe Newburg, BRNC*

Variation: This same five-senses approach can be applied to a season, holiday, favorite or least favorite day of the week, etc.

MONDAY

Monday is red because everything begins;
It sounds soft and whispery;
It has the good smell and taste of everything cooking;
Monday feels smooth and makes me feel good —

When I first wake up on Monday morning,
I wonder who will help me dress —
And I like it that everything is beginning on TV!

—Vanetta Bealle, BRNC

My least favorite day used to be Monday —
Monday was washday in our house;
My mother would go around
Gathering up the things to be washed
And nine times out of ten, I'd be wearing
Something that just had to be washed!
Monday would have to be blue;
It sounds like "Swish-swish";
It smells fetid and damp;
It tastes like cucumber — I can't bear them!
Monday is rough like sandpaper!

—Joan Brindley, BRNC

4. What We Have Loved

The five senses can help turn what might otherwise be just a list
of things loved over a lifetime into a vivid, involving poem. An
excellent inspiration is Rubert Brooke's poem, "The Great Lover,"
particularly the part starting "These I have loved:" and ending with
"All these have been my loves," because his sensory images are
superb and he uses alliteration effectively.
   Guidelines:

— Read the Brooke and other example poems.
— Talk about the vividness of the images — ask the group which
  were their favorites; point out the wide variety of the images
  and the way they contrast with each other and give the poem
  energy.
— Summarize on the tablet: "What have *you* loved in your lifetime? Choose at least one sight, one sound, one taste, one
  texture, one smell. Describe each as vividly as possible and
  put them together in a poem, saving your strongest or most
  surprising image for the last line."

Examples:

THESE I HAVE LOVED
Feeling scratchy sandpaper
When making something in shop;
Smelling flowers in
The hot air of August;
Looking at the white
Blanketed trees in the
Cold, crisp air of winter;
Seeing happy faces;
Hearing running water or
Watching rain fall;
Listening to the radio
In my nice, warm, soft bed
Covered with a silky,
Cotton, warm blanket.

—Wendy Peck, Grade 5

These I have loved all through the years,
Feelings that bring both laughter and tears:
The view from the top of Clingman's Dome
With the winding road leading home;
The running brook tumbling over the rocks,
The visits of friends who come and knock;
The bright sun coloring the west
Before a quiet evening of rest;
The melodious sounds of the organ on Sunday morning,
Looking forward to a new week dawning;
There is no end to love
In earth below or heaven above.

—Marie Huff, BRNC

These I have loved—
The shine of silk upon someone moving,
The sound of a French horn in a symphony orchestra,
The smell of chili sauce wafting through the house
        in the days when we used to "put up" things;

The taste of a hot fudge sundae when I'd donated my money
    to the local store
  instead of to the church collection plate;
The soft wooly feel of my white angora sweater—
  how my date hated that sweater when he was wearing
  his best black suit!

—Joan Brindley, BRNC

These I have loved—
The people in the poetry group,
The sound of music and poetry,
The smell of lilies of the valley—
They tell you a lot of things.

—Helen Shoemaker, BRNC

These I have loved—
The sounds of people being busy,
The color yellow,
The smell of clean, pure air,
The feel of my soft shawl.

—Sarah McInteer, BRNC

These things I have loved to see—
Antique garnets on pale pink satin,
A lofty street lamp smothered in fog,
A small child coping with a large caterpillar,
Or a madly paislied red quilt tossed free
  on a snow white sheet;
I have loved sound like the
Beloved call that claims, "I'm home!"
Or the beautiful quiet that follows a toned down noise
And the gorgeously spaced clutter of Bach;
I love all tastes that my mouth can assume,
And the textures of these are well woven into the memories
that I own and keep for myself.

—Helen L. Anderson, BRNC

5. What We've Known

In "The Negro Speaks of Rivers," Langston Hughes shows his people's deep attachment to rivers by speaking as if he were personally involved to the point of feeling part of them. The imagery is simple but powerful. The writing idea is to describe something you've known so well that you have sometimes felt part of it, to let your vivid images *show* your involvement without your having to tell it.

Guidelines:

— Read example poems and enjoy the imagery together.
— Summarize idea on the tablet: "Think of something you've known well during your life — in nature, manmade, an activity, a place, an art, a food, even a feeling. Show your involvement with it, your feelings about it through vivid description. Try to build to a strong ending."

Examples:

I'VE KNOWN MOUNTAINS

I've known mountains —
Tall steep slopes with big boulders;
I've climbed Mount Jefferson and I touched
Each breath of wind that flew past;
I've gathered every grain of soil,
Every rock and flake of snow for Mr. Everest;
I've swooped over Mr. Washington with the high, howling winds;
My soul jumped over the Himalayas and came back to me
And told me all the beautiful things;
My body feels close to all the different mountains.

— Kate Brown, Grade 3

I'VE KNOWN THE SUN

I've known the sun —
I feel like I'm part of it;
I threw planets out into orbits;
I burn people on the beach;

I made people go insane on deserts;
I helped the planets grow into suns
To reflect them;
I shine over the ice and make a
Blinding light;
I showed the Viking how to navigate;
I keep Solarex in business;
I make it so people on earth can be warm;
I've always been the center of the
Universe;
I and the sun are one.

—Paul DeLaney, Grade 4

I've known the Chesapeake Bay—
Over fifty years I have been using it as my second bathtub
And have seen man change it from spring water to sewage;
I have swum the mile from our shore to Baltimore shore,
Which is now an international airport;
The hum of mosquitos and the croaking of bullfrogs
Make good company every evening;
The frogs and mosquitos and trees
Make unbeatable nighttime companions;
The hum of the boats has changed
From Metro Station to a natural, placid state;
It's built up so that I can't use the boat any more,
But I know the Chesapeake Bay.

—Dorothy Ahrens, BRNC

I've known flowers—
I've lain dormant in the ground,
Waiting for the first sign of warm spring sunshine;
I've emitted my perfume to the air;
I've felt little fuzzy humming animals drinking of my nectar;
I've helped make a young girl blush with pride;
I've been tossed by a young bride to someone else;
I've also at times been on the other end
And have been tossed onto a casket;
Ah, yes—I've known flowers!

—Joan Brindley, BRNC

B. NEW VISIONS OF THE FAMILIAR

Metaphor is one of a poet's best friends, adding life and zest to writing by showing similarities between seemingly unlike things. When I work with very young children I usually tell them that I'm going to show them how to use their "new eyes." With older groups, I translate the word into its two Greek roots ("meta" = "across" and "phor" = "carry") and mention that if the comparison is obvious, such as "clouds are fluffy cotton," the metaphor is not going to be as strong as if it surprises and, as a result, delights the reader—for example, "a marshmallow is an albino ant with elephantiasis," as my son wrote in fifth grade. Although I encourage students to make comparisons without using "like" or "as," some are simply more comfortable with similes, such as Robert Burns' "My love is like a red, red rose," so I don't fuss at them. And a few of the writing projects, like (2) below, just seem naturally to turn out as similes.

1. New Eyes On Ourselves

In this project, writers give new views of themselves through metaphors comparing themselves to particular animals, flowers, books, houses, musical instruments, colors, tools, cars, trees, jewelry, birds, fruits, vegetables, desserts, letters, numbers, geometric shapes, furniture, machines, etc. It is easy to introduce the idea by asking, "Have you ever thought of yourself as an animal? Which one? Why?" Or "What flower would you say you are like? Why?" It is fun to compare notes informally before writing.
Guidelines:

— Read several example poems, pointing out that the poets compare themselves to a wide variety of things and show why they are like them.
— Write the pattern on the big tablet: "I am a _____ because _____" and stress that the "because" part is as important as the metaphor.
— Make a list of many different categories of things they might use but of course are not restricted to, such as those listed above.

—Summarize the directions: "Write at least five metaphors comparing yourself to different things and telling why; then arrange them into a poem that is your metaphoric self-portrait—remember to choose a *variety* of things and to build up to your best one at the end."

Variations:

a. One time I prepared a "fill-in" sheet of about ten lines following the form "I am a (specific tool) because _____" and included a space for writing a poem based on one or more of the metaphors; some people expanded a single metaphor into a terrific poem.

b. Another time I chose the category and had everyone write an expanded metaphor on "What Flower Are You?" I suspect that "house" would work well, too.

c. Another time I used the "conditional" approach—"If I were a _____ I would be _____ because . . ."

d. Still another time I used the basic comparison idea to focus on feelings: "When I am angry (or happy, lonely, frustrated, etc.) I am like a _____." When using this approach it is best to make a long list of various feelings on the tablet and copy the pattern. This writing idea has been around for such a long time that I do not know its original source.

e. Another possibility would be to use Kenneth Koch's idea, in *Wishes, Lies and Dreams*, of pairing "I used to be a _____, But now I am a _____" and possibly adding "I wish I were a _____."

Examples:

METAPHORIC ME!

I am a dolphin because I am sleek;
I am a root because I grow with my family;
I am a computer because I play games;
I am numbers four and twenty-eight because I am not odd;
I am a Porsche because I am fast;
I am gold and silver because I am rich with laughter.

—Adam Vine, Grade 2

METAPHORIC ME!

I am a valley; I run in the wild.
I am a ballet shoe; I spin around.
I am a broom; I sweep people off their feet.
I am a book; I am full of entertainment.
I am a ruler; people ask me how old I am.
I am an air conditioner; I am always cool.
I am the sun; I burst with glee!

—Greer Boyle, Grade 4

I am a sponge because I soak up ideas, impressions and thoughts
    from everything around me;
I am a bowl in which I stir all that my mind contains;
I am a judge selecting what I want to retain and from which I
    weave
My own pattern for life.

—Dorothy Yates—BRNC

I am like a daisy because I like the sun;
I am like spring, filled with sunshine;
I am like Wednesday, right in the middle of things!
I am like yellow, very happy.

—Sarah McInteer, BRNC

I am a horse because I like to run fast;
I am a piano because I like to play;
I am a pink African violet because I bloom all day;
I am a pair of scissors because I can do things and I am sharp;
I am a teddy bear because I like to cuddle;
I am a book of poetry because I *like* poetry;
I am nearly white like the flower on my bureau because that's
    what I am!

I am a big house with a fireplace because that's where I used
    to live.

                              —Vanetta Bealle, BRNC

(Variation A)

I am like a piano — filled with classical music;
I have my own language and many keys to my personality;
I have different parts and things inside me
    that don't show on the outside;
No two pianos are alike.

                              —Laura Bonesteel, BRNC

I was a tree one lifetime —
That was the time I got used to what they called weather;
I was a fir tree and lived in New England;
I used to shake my branches and laugh at weather —
Hot or cold I could take it.
What amused me the most was people
Talking about the hot summer and the cold winters!

                              —Dorothy Emerson, BRNC

I am a soup kettle hanging by a hook
    on the far side of a door to the closet
Where things not often used are safely away
    but available when needed.
I am dented by falls and scratched by scrubbing
But polished well — even over the bumpy black reminders
    of over-eager flames.
My usefulness has never been questioned,
But success has varied,
Particularly when my lid was not on straight
    or needed a new handle on top.
But I still have the capacity for a marvelous stew
    or a soup of stature —
So long as ingredients are generously tossed
I can still produce a worthy broth
That has nothing to do with my age!

                              —Helen L. Anderson, BRNC

(Variation B)

WHAT FLOWER AM I?

The geranium—
It can adapt itself to all kinds of temperatures;
Sunshine it likes and it thrives if it gets enough;
It can stand winds and all kinds of adversaries,
As I had to learn to do.
I want to be the flower of a linden tree,
Smelling very sweet, opening up in spring,
Helping people to get well when they have a cold,
Being useful to others.

—Anna Goldschmidt, BRNC

I am baby's breath—
It looks weak and delicate
But it's strong;
It lasts a long time
And goes well with other flowers;
You can grow it anywhere
And it fits.

—Betty Graham, BRNC

(Variation C)

I'd like to be the color blue
Because it's the color of the sky
And the color of the ocean, too;
I'd like to be cool and refreshing
To other people.

—Catherine J. Curtin, BRNC

I'd like to be yellow—it's so cheerful
And there's so much gloom everywhere—
Gloomy things, gloomy people.
If I were an animal I'd like to be a fish—
A fish can swim all day, eat all day, see beautiful scenery all day;
Then again—a fish can be eaten by another fish!

If I were a musical instrument I'd like to be a harp —
Any practice I could get in this world would make me
    more acceptable in the next, providing I went up, not down.
If I were a tool I'd like to be a plane —
Sometimes I'd leave strips of wood and sometimes I'd leave
    curls.
If I were a flower I'd like to be a sunflower —
My face would turn to the sun and birds would love my seeds —
    humans, too.
If I were a tree there would be no choice for me —
I'd definitely be a weeping willow;
They are so graceful with their long skirts sweeping the ground,
And every once in a while the wind would come along and help.
I wouldn't want to be any darn book I know of!
Many people use books to press flowers or to reach the high
    shelf,
And some books are left in private libraries, to gather dust.
If I were an object I'd like to be a bookend —
Just think, every time I held my stomach in,
A whole bunch of people would fall down!

—*Joan Brindley, BRNC*

(Variation D)

FEELINGS ALIVE!

When I am happy, I am like a butterfly;
When I am angry, I am like thunder;
When I am sad, I am like a leaf that is rotted;
When I am excited, I am like a very strange hyena;
When I am lonely, I am like a bird on a gate;
When I am tired, I am like a rag doll;
When I am crazy, I am like a blizzard;
When I am itchy, I am like a baby monkey;
When I am embarrassed, I am like a hiding kitten;
When I am ambitious, I am like a dog looking for a bone;
When I am loving, I am like a cuddly panda.

—*Mary Dowling, Grade 2*

When I am happy, I'm like a bunny hopping through the tall
    green grass;
When I am excited, I'm like a balloon with its air pouring out;
When I am mad, I am like a pot full of liver;
When I am left out, I feel like the only green leaf on the tree;
When I am tired, I feel like the clouds floating through the sky.

                —Rebecca Crocker, Grade 4

When I am happy I am like a dog getting a bone;
When I am angry I am like a cat meeting a dog;
When I am sad I am like the moon that's vanishing;
When I am excited I am like very loud music playing.
When I am tired I am like a wrung out piece of dishcloth;
When I am bored I am like a sleeping child;
When I am embarrassed I am like meeting an old foe;
When I am grumpy I am like the old, cold winter;
When I am surprised I am like being asked to marry my beloved;
When I am lonely I am like a house whose inhabitants moved;
When I am loving I am like a bird in spring;
When I am busy I am like a writer ending a book;
When I am lazy I am like a child that's tired;
When I am moody I am like an angry cat or the weather before
    a storm.

                —Anna Goldschmidt, BRNC

When I am lonely I am like a tree
Standing by itself in a big field;
When I am happy I am like a laughing family—
I just feel grateful that my family are
Coming along on good lines and doing so well;
As long as the kids are happy
I have no right to feel unhappy about anything.

                —Ethel Boesch, BRNC

2. New Visions of Other People

In this project we turn our new eyes on other people in general or those we know best in particular, comparing them to specific items in a general classification, such as shoes, jewelry, cars, trees, books, foods, etc. and show why they are like that.

Guidelines:

- — After presenting the idea of comparing people to things nonhuman, and showing what they have in common, make a list on the tablet of many different categories the writers might consider — "animals," "plants," "trees," "colors," "houses," "tools," "clothing," "shoes," "foods," "jewelry," "furniture," "books," "musical instruments," "machines," "vehicles," etc., much like the list for Project 1 above.
- — Emphasize that they are to link specific people, such as people in their families, people in the nursing home, people who fill different roles, with specifics within the category chosen and to show why the comparison is accurate.
- — Summarize on the tablet: "Choose one category and a group of people with which to compare it. In your poem, compare specific people to specific items within the category, and show why, using the form (specific person) is like (specific item) because _____. You may use any other form that works for you."

Examples:

PEOPLE ARE LIKE SHOES

My father is like a pair of penny loafers because
He's always full of money, but he never wants to spend it.
My sister is like a pair of sneakers because
She is tough, rugged and can handle almost anything.
I am like a pair of ballet shoes because
I get worn out.
My mother is like a pair of Jellies because
She's flexible, soft, nice,
Not too warm, not too cold, but just right.

—Leslie Davis, Grade 3

PEOPLE ARE LIKE STONES

My mother is like a bright and shiny one
   because she is lively and never quiet;
My dad is an old one
   because he knows nearly everything;
My sister is a soft one
   because she learns easily;
My little brother is gold
   because he is worth a lot and he shines;
My other brother is a diamond
   because he is stubborn and will not let you
   tell him anything.

—Rob Johnston, Grade 4

PEOPLE ARE LIKE PAPER

My sister is like a roll of paper towels—rough and always out
   of it when I am around;
My mom is like a piece of school paper—always strict and neat;
My dad is like a roll of Charmin—always soft and big
   and huggable;
My teachers are like bright colors of paper—always full of fun
   and excitement;
My friends are like a piece of drawing paper—always there
   when you need it;
My grandma is like a paper bag—always full of good gifts
   and plentiful.

—Sara Hayes, Grade 3

PEOPLE ARE LIKE BOOKS

Books have paper or board bindings,
People have legs, arms and heads;
Individually each is different—
People speak various dialects,
Books are written in many different languages;
Books and people have a message for the world—
Some are good, some evil,

Some are spiritual, some worldly;
Each leaves a mark as it passes through life,
And so the wealth of knowledge
Builds through generations and centuries.

—Dorothy Yates, BRNC

My husband Luther was like a diamond and sapphire necklace—
He always glittered but not in a showy way;
He was genuine throughout;
I adored the ground he walked on;
He brought happiness and joy to many with his voice
And brought beauty into my life for forty-six years;
He was a gem—no doubt about that—
Best of all, both he and the necklace belonged to me.

—Alice Balliet, BRNC

PEOPLE ARE LIKE THE ROOMS OF A HOUSE

At BRNC, Mrs. Grey-Coker, Mrs. Symes, Mrs. Conlin and Mrs.
   Clay are like a library—they are full of knowledge like the
   books of the library and they are also very comforting like the
   easy chairs and attractive divans one finds in well-furnished
   libraries;
Mrs. Lee is a violin from the music room, playing bright happy
   music for all the staff;
Beckie and Geri are a lovely family room where everyone is
   welcome—their many offerings of music, art, crafts, games,
   movies, and reading matter of all sorts—surely every member
   of the BRNC family can find something interesting there;
Brenda and Mary are the room, so pretty and cheerful, where
   everyone goes in search of the body beautiful;
Mrs. Manuel and Mrs. Wines are the entrance to the house,
   directing with charm and efficiency the entire structure;
Frank is the electric switch that makes everything work;
Mrs. Connor is Hebe, bearing wine from room to room, not to
   gods but to grateful mortals;
Mrs. Long is the heart of the house with her kitchen, where
   marvelous food is produced.

—Vida Hickerson, BRNC

3. Weather Creatures

This idea is based on Carl Sandburg's well-known little poem "Fog." Many people will know it, but it is short enough to copy in big letters onto a large piece of paper and bring in so everyone can see. I usually ask the group why they think Sandburg chose a cat for comparison with fog, and they enjoy pointing out all the similarities. The writing project is to choose any kind of weather and compare it to an animal, considering the animal's appearance, movements, personality, general behavior, etc.

Guidelines:

— Brainstorm with the class for all the kinds of weather they can think of and list them on the tablet.
— Brainstorm for a wide variety of animals and list them on the tablet.
— List the animal specifics to consider: appearance (including skin or fur, eyes, teeth, tail, feet, body, etc.), personality (i.e., furtive and sneaky or gregarious), and especially movements—it helps to list several verbs that show movement, such as "leap," "sneak," "slither," "jump," "glide," "lumber," "thump," "stalk," "pad," "tiptoe," "scamper," "hop," "amble," "prance," "gallop," "soar," "swoop," "totter," etc.
— Summarize idea: "Choose a weather condition and write about it as if it were an animal—show how it arrives, how it looks, how it moves, how it leaves—be as specific and vivid as possible."

Examples:

WIND

Wind roars in like a lion over the countryside;
The paw of the lion swats down leaves
And sometimes even trees if the lion is mad—
That is called a hurricane;
When the lion gets tired, the wind stops;
Then the small cubs make a cool summer breeze.

—Phillip Kronstein, Grade 2

SUN

The sun flies down as a canary would
His wings are golden yellow;
His wings are as soft as a canary feather;
His nest is as golden as his wings.

—Chris Ziener, Grade 3

A STORM WITH ANIMALS

The lightning in the dark night is a yellow panther
Jumping down from the night sky;
The rain is the panther's saliva
Dripping down from his mouth;
When he eats, the storm cloud is his breath;
The thunder is when he stamps in the clouds;
The panther is heavy, and when he jumps on a tree,
It breaks.

—Fielding Ince, Grade 3

STORM

The storm is a gray panther:
He starts out quiet,
Then all of the sudden
He drops—
He is wild—
He makes everybody know who is boss;
He shrieks and howls—
He wants you to know
He can do all kinds of things,
Ripping and tearing,
Showing where he has been;
You always have to know he was there—
He makes it so you remember him!
The whole universe is upset!

—Dorothy Oest, BRNC

SNOWSTORM

Great snowstorms are like polar bears
Seeking lost cubs:

Huge moving whitened masses
Filling the frigid emptiness
With the sound of eager searching,
Offering the embracing white fur like
Protection that covers both
Lost and found alike
And after the force of the action, leaving
A soothing sense of wondrous maternal care!

—Helen L. Anderson, BRNC

STORM

A storm is a busy little spider —
It minds its own business for a while,
But before you know it,
You're caught up in its web
And everything shakes like it's coming apart;
But after it passes and the sun comes out,
Everything glistens like a jewel;
Except for a few repairs here and there,
Everything is the same.

—Joan Brindley, BRNC

Variation: Feeling Creatures. Instead of weather, compare a feeling to a creature, again showing how it looks and moves, arrives and leaves.

LOVE

Love is a bird, wings of forgiveness, seeds of hearts, caring, and sliding ever so softly through the wind, seeing that everybody reproduces. In one place there is fighting, hatred, and anger, but once it gets there, there is love like once before. It is slow, it is gentle, it never hurts anybody! Every night at midnight the bird digs underground to the sun which is her nest, and in the morning it's gliding through the air ever so softly.

—Megan Wallace, Grade 3

HATRED, THE SCORPION

Hatred is a scorpion,
Always getting you by surprise,
Lashing up from one place
   when you expect it from somewhere else,
Stinging and swelling,
Making you do things
   you normally wouldn't do.
The scorpion has glowing eyes,
   sharp teeth, scaly and rough skin,
     spiny legs and stinging tail.
It lives inside you,
Stinging you and making you
   lash out and hurt other people.
It swallows the little joy
   so all that is left is Hatred.
It kills all happiness with
   one lash of its deadly tail,
But sometimes happiness kills it —
Then it dies down,
   only to strike again.
It fears happiness, joy,
   love and friendship.

— Theresa Bradley, Grade 4

Joy is a hummingbird
With its ruby throat and bright wings
Always on the move,
Darting here, then far off,
Seeking nectar in flowers,
Shunning dull, tasteless objects,
Never quiet, never satisfied,
But giving joy to all who see it.

— Dorothy Yates, BRNC

Joy is a lizard
That keeps jumping up in the air;
It likes sunlight and moves very quickly

From one person to another
And lives in a hidden place.

— *Vanetta Bealle, BRNC*

Grief is a condor functioning loftily alone,
Beautifully patterned against the mountain reverted sky,
Its hooded search seeking out and joying only in
The spoilage and demise of what once lived;
But when this ugliness departs all fatly sated,
It leaves in such wing-fluttering splendor
That its regal departure becomes
Almost exquisite to behold!

— *Helen L. Anderson, BRNC*

4. New Eyes On Food

One of my most popular projects with all age groups is looking at familiar foods in a new way and writing metaphors to show those new visions. Three foods that work very well, and that usually everyone can eat, are popcorn, marshmallows, and "regular" size Fritos. The first time I did this, I passed out all three items, but for subsequent times, I used just one at a time. One Thanksgiving I read them the story in *Childcraft* about how the Indians introduced the Pilgrims to popcorn at the first Thanksgiving feast and then asked them to look at popcorn in a new way. I have also used grapefruit, bananas, and a fresh pineapple in the middle of the table.

Guidelines:

— Tell everyone that you are going to write about something very familiar, even ordinary, but that they are going to look at it with new eyes and see the extraordinary in it.
— Hold up a piece of popcorn (or a marshmallow or a Frito) and ask what their "old eyes" see — then say something like, "But when you look at it with your new eyes, you might see a soft tooth with a large cavity, or a Barbie doll's brain, or a tiny white cobra tied up in knots or the Jolly Green Giant's dandruff!"

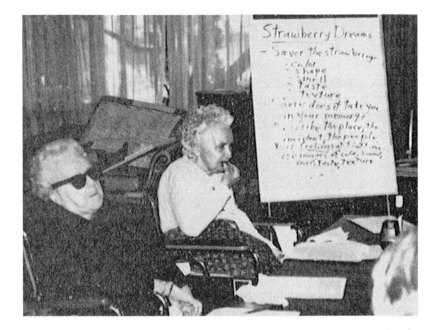

Alice Balliet thinks about the poem she will dictate, and Eleanor O'Brien savors her strawberry.

Photo by Wendy C. Webster.

— Pass out a handful of popcorn (or a marshmallow or a few Fritos) and a napkin to each person.
— On the large tablet write: "'What do your new eyes see in the popcorn (or marshmallow or Frito)?' Think of it as something giant or something miniature, perhaps. Write metaphors about what you see, following the form, 'Popcorn is. . . . . . .' Try for a wide variety of metaphors, and put them in their best dramatic order."

Examples:

Popcorn is . . .
A dehydrated sponge tied in the middle,
An ivory white frog with seedy eyes,

A bloated tadpole,
Petrified whipped cream,
A bleached rooster,
A flower born of violence.

— High School workshop

Popcorn is . . .
A jellyfish with spots,
A broken ballerina chopped in half,
A hat for an ant.

— Brian Herrmann, Grade 1

Popcorn is . . .
An explosion of white and brown,
A pure white hill muddied by a skier,
A white hat with a brown ribbon,
White gloves in a big, dirty city,
White pearls on brown thread,
Immature animals of the Sargasso Sea,
   waiting to be gobbled up so some other animal can grow.

— Joan Brindley, BRNC

Popcorn is music —
It blooms from the inside,
Surprising you with its sound and shape,
And makes you feel good inside;
When it is gone
It is a beautiful memory.

— Catherine J. Curtin, BRNC

Popcorn looks like a hard pillow covered by a case;
It is cut from the cob and dried;
I think of it when it pops!
And the only thing I don't like about it is
I can eat every bit of it that's put in front of me!
It also looks like cotton batting that got wet!

— Margaret T. Edwards, BRNC

Popcorn looks like personalities of people which we so often find
Quite pure and white on the outside,
Covering a little brown spot on the inside
That is neither good to look at or follow in any way;
Therefore I think that perhaps
The lovely white purity on the outside
Makes us want to cover up the brown part;
If we can think of white popcorn
Covering up the nonedible brown spot,
Perhaps we can think of the good in personalities
And not the bad spots.

—Laura Bonesteel, BRNC

A marshmallow is . . .
A wedding cake for doves,
A love boat for powder,
Silklike clouds unable to rain,
A pillow for a butterfly,
A soft, rubber cloud,
A roll of Charmin for some grasshoppers,
A guinea pig's drum.

— 4th grade workshop

A marshmallow is . . .
A fluffy bed for an ant!
Or a nice pillow for a cricket!
Or a rainbow that got stuck in a cloud!

—Jamie Hechinger, Grade 2

A marshmallow is . . .
The milk of the milkweed all bunched together;
A tiny white ball rolling in the sand;
A wheel of the car of a cricket.

—Phoebe Johnson, Grade 2

A Frito is . . .
Petrified Scotch tape,

A steam-rollered worm,
A hand-knit scarf boiled in hot suds,
A warped magic carpet after dry cleaning,
A toothless old clam,
A rhinoceros's toenail,
A clam shell closed for the day,
A wilted sultan's slipper.

— Teacher workshop

Popcorn is a torn bag;
A Frito is a snake's tongue;
A marshmallow is a doll's hat;
A marshmallow is a dish full of ice cream;
A Frito is a dying worm;
Popcorn is a crumpled piece of paper;
Popcorn is a snake turning around.

—Anna Goldschmidt, BRNC

A marshmallow is a stool I sat on;
Popcorn is a little cat I had —
He was snow white and always slept at the foot of my bed;
He was named Peter;
If there was no one at home, I could always talk to Peter,
For he knew every word I said.

—Florence Canning, BRNC

NEW EYES ON GRAPEFRUIT

A yellow object — what is it?
A ball for playing games?
A rounded daub of dough?
A blob of mud?
Cut it open and the beauty of
Rich fruit appears;
A wealth of flavor awaits
The explorer;
A treasure chest of gold is his.

—Dorothy Yates, BRNC

NEW EYES ON BANANAS

A banana makes me think
Of a swing on a hot summer's day
Being swung between two shade trees;
It also makes me see the boats in Hawaii
With a man standing up at the rear, guiding;
It is a precious food to eat!

—Louise Oldenbusch, BRNC

A PINEAPPLE IS . . .

A geyser frozen in midair,
A million stars dancing around a tree,
Pins in a hard pincushion,
A rocket taking off with green exhaust,
Snakes coming out of a sack,
Peacock eyes wrapped around a palm tree,
A turtle with a crewcut,
A short-haired porcupine with a long bushy tail,
A frightened person with hair straight up,
Green fire from an orange torch!

—5th grade workshop

PINEAPPLE

Pineapple makes me think of happiness!
It looks like a little house
I built for the children—
It was all happiness!

—Lillian Dorrance, BRNC

PINEAPPLE

I can remember when we were in Hawaii
And saw fields of pineapple—
They looked like little palm trees.
They would let us help ourselves—
We would take them home and eat them—
They were most delicious!

They tasted like the most refreshing drink.
You could play tic-tac-toe on the skin!

—Louise Oldenbusch, BRNC

A PINEAPPLE

It looks like a flower pot with fancy paper around
And a plant on top;
It feels like a grating iron bothering my hand;
It would say, "Taste me";
It reminds me of my mother's appreciation for its taste,
And it reminds me of the cheap canned pineapple
We got in London at the start of the war.
P.S. It looks like a porcupine with a dozen heads.

—Anna Goldschmidt, BRNC

Variation: New Eyes on Geometry. Ask the writers to look at familiar shapes, such as the circle and the square, see them with new vision and write metaphors to show what they have seen. Remind them about a variety of images and a good progression for them.

Examples:

NEW EYES ON A CIRCLE

A circle is the world:
It is a carriage wheel spinning,
It is a calm lake at sunset,
It is a stomach growling,
It is a clock chiming,
It is a glass of warm milk,
It is a can of frozen orange juice,
It is a marble rolling around,
It is an eye looking at you,
It is a zero in the number 10.

—Tim Paster, Grade 2

CIRCLES

A circle is the moon,
   throwing showers of light to earth;
A tortoise shell, as the huge animal
   goes plodding slowly forward;
The bottom of an elephant's foot,
   crushing its dinner of hay;
A pearl, just sitting there inside the oyster,
   disturbing no one, only waiting
   to be pulled out;
A lonely stump, giving a tired old traveler
   a place to rest;
A circle of love, growing bigger and bigger
   as each new person in the world makes friends.

—Amanda Whitehead, Grade 3

ABOUT CIRCLES

I feel that there is
An awful lot of thinking going on
But not passed on to the next one —
I circulate,
But my thoughts don't.

— Ethel Boesch, BRNC

A circle·can be a whole bunch of things —
It can be a line that turned away from being a straight line,
A wedding ring,
The sun coming up;
You're so glad you have the circle to write about —
You just look at it
And hope you get something decent from it —
It can be anything!

— Dorothy Oest, BRNC

A circle is a roundabout story.

—Ralph M. Prouty, BRNC

An empty circle is a new life
Waiting to be colored in.
With each one comes a pail of paint
And a wide brush, freshly clean;
We are warned to fill it in
And not beyond the edge;
We madly splatter, spill and spray,
Make rare designs and adverse angles,
    loops and twirls
And slither off the side;
But few of us live long enough
To fill its simple form.

— Helen L. Anderson, BRNC

NEW EYES ON TRIANGLES

A triangle reminds me of
A piece of leaf
Or of cheese
Or a pyramid.

— Sarah McInteer, BRNC

A triangle takes you to the Statue of Liberty via the Staten
    Island Ferry;
I think the Ferry is still a nickel —
You could do all sorts of things on the 5-cent ride, like games;
We had to take turns riding on the Ferry when I was young.

— Judith Weinman, BRNC

5. Transformations

Another way to look at ourselves differently and reveal our personalities is to turn ourselves imaginatively into wind, rain, snow, clouds, the sun, the moon, stars, etc. and describe our appearance and behavior. I have often linked this assignment to the weather outside — it is sometimes easier and more fun to imagine being snow when the season's first is falling outside.

Guidelines:

— Ask the group if they have ever imagined what it would be like
   to be snow (or wind, rain, a cloud, the moon, or whatever) and
   trade a few ideas about things they could do or places they
   could go that people cannot.
— Write leading questions on the tablet: "If you were snow, how
   would you look? How would you feel? How would you move?
   How would you sound? Where would you live? What would
   you do all day? Who would your friends be? Where would you
   go on vacation? What would you dream about at night?"
— Remind them to be as specific as possible and to build up to a
   good ending.

Examples:

IF I WERE SNOW

If I were snow
I would flutter down in the wind
And touch the ground and lie stiffly;
I would feel round and cold;
I would feel the metal on the snow shovel;
I would dream about melting on the ground;
I'd smell clean and wet;
I'd move softly against the wind;
My favorite place would be on a roof
With a bunch of other snowflakes;
I would taste like clear water in the summer;
I would sound like a light breeze.

— Emily Brunner, Kindergarten

IF I WERE SNOW . . .
Quietly falling earthward
I would cover trees and fields
With a warm, soft blanket
White and unmarred,
Making a slate
For the tracks of all living creatures,
A record of a day's activities.

— Dorothy Yates, BRNC

If I were snow
I would try to resume my original state;
I could form a solid mass which would
Eventually become a large white house —
A house without snow people?
Furniture? A kitchen, fully supplied with appliances?
A large attractively painted sign reading somewhat as follows —
"Lovely home for a couple of snow people
And their flaky little ones."

—Judith Weinman, BRNC

Were I a snowflake
Not burdened by wisdom of age
   or well-known facts,
I'd dance a wild search
For what does not exist —
A perfect match for me!

—Helen L. Anderson, BRNC

BEING WIND

I'm a wind that blows the feathers on birds,
I talk cool to the sun!
Sometimes when I go to the playground with children,
I make their hair fly up;
I live in the attic of heaven.

—Ashleigh Davis, Kindergarten

If I were the wind I would shatter the windowpanes
And make the little crosses on the windows crooked;
I'd sound like somebody blowing;
My friend would be the sun;
I'd eat leaves from trees;
On vacation I'd go to South America.

—Morley McBride, Kindergarten

If I were the wind
I'd find lots of funny things,
Blow a particular lady's hat off;
I'd probably have my face slapped,
So I'd have to go away,
Lord only knows where!
I'm lost up in the trees, just now,
And they can't seem to find me!
I think I'll take it rather easy —
I'm getting rather old, now!

— Ethel Boesch, BRNC

If I were the wind I would sweep flower seeds all over;
I would blow so strong in a tornado to frighten everyone,
And sometimes I would blow soft,
Just helping the ships come into port,
Like Richard Wagner says in "The Flying Dutchman."
I would complain that the sun is too hot;
I would brag about my power to frighten everybody;
I would bring such chilling weather that rivers froze,
Bragging about my power to freeze the rivers.
In early spring I would blow softly and be careful
Not to blow blooming plant blossoms off too quickly.

— Anna Goldschmidt, BRNC

BEING A CLOUD

If I were a cloud
I would rain on people;
I would get a stomach ache
    when planes went through me;
I would be friends with the sun;
I would make hail;
I would go to the sea and get some steam;
I would snow on people;
I would make a rainbow in the sky;
I would make warm weather;
I would make a storm;
I would go to Saturn;

I would make it cold;
I would make a mackerel cloud.

—Ashley Wivel, Grade 2

IF I WERE A CLOUD . . .

I'd be a hurricane cloud;
I'd step right up and get to work;
Of course, being a cloud,
I'd have so much strength
I'd get to work on all the clouds below me
And make my presence felt;
I'd look threatening (but not to me);
I'd be so glad I could scare everybody!
I'd feel happy I had so much power!
I'd scare everybody good—
I'd be not too smart, but I'd do that!

—Dorothy Oest, BRNC

IF I WERE A CLOUD . . .

I would look dark and cold;
I would swoop down on people
And make them miserable;
I would feel cold and sticky;
I would visit stars and the moon;
I would fly over the sky.

—Betty Graham, BRNC

C. FORMS AND ORGANIZING FORCES

I would not advise introducing long, complicated, or terribly restrictive forms, as some class members become confused, frustrated and discouraged, especially those who have never written poetry before joining the group. But working within a set framework or under the discipline of an organizing force can be a good experience, a particular kind of triumph. I have had the most success with Acrostics, short Oriental forms, Recipes, and some organizing structures borrowed from professional poets.

1. Acrostics

In this form, the poet writes the subject of the poem *vertically* beside the lefthand margin. Each letter becomes the initial letter of the first word in that line, which describes the subject in some way. Some poets add the restriction that every word in the line, such as a series of adjectives or verbs, must begin with that letter. This is a good form to use when writing about a holiday or season and is especially good for people's names — a self-portrait.

Guidelines:

- It is best to introduce this by demonstration on a big tablet. Write your subject in large letters down the left edge of the paper and ask the group for descriptive words that begin with each letter. You could take the time to do two, showing both ways of approaching it.
- As always, remind the writers to search for the most vivid words for their poems.

Examples:

Smells of fall,
Every bird and bee sounds stronger,
Powerful smells of crops getting old,
The leaves changing to gold and ochre,
Elegance everywhere,
Moon turns autumn-colored,
Beginning of fall,
Everything tastes like fall,
Ripe pears are juicy and good.

— Betty Graham, BRNC

Summer is passing,
Emptying the branches,
Pulling the blooms to earth,
Taking back the riches

Enjoyed all summer;
Memory will keep them fresh,
Bringing back the beauty
Enjoyed all summer;
Remember, remember until spring comes.

—Dorothy Yates, BRNC

Cards, carols, cheer, chestnuts, cold
Horses (that's what used to pull the sleighs)
Ruin (many people go into financial ruin at Xmas)
Ink (it's what you're supposed to use when signing cards)
Snow
Time (will Christmas *ever* get here?)
Money (it takes a lot of this around Xmas)
Aunt (wonder what *she'll* send this year?)
Santa (of course)

—Joan Brindley, BRNC

A TRIBUTE TO OUR NURSES

Nourish our needs,
Usually come quickly to a call,
Reassure us when we are troubled,
Soothe our pains,
Entirely dedicated to those in pain,
Smile and say kind words in dark hours.

—Group poem for the BRNC nurses

2. Oriental Forms

The Japanese haiku has been a popular form to use with students of all ages for a number of years, now, and there are several good books on the subject. My class at the nursing home has also enjoyed some lesser known oriental forms, such as the tanka and the cinquain (reputedly an early form of the haiku, but there is some question).

a. Tanka

This form, most popular in the tenth, eleventh and twelfth centuries, was known for being the court poetry of Japan's golden age. Before Japan had a written language people recited tanka, and they are still written today. Every year the Emperor sponsors a tanka contest. Like the haiku, it has a specific number of syllables in each line, but it has five instead of only three lines. The lines are arranged: 5 syllables, 7 syllables, 5 syllables, 7 syllables, 7 syllables. As far as I know, it is not limited to nature, as is the haiku, but as with the haiku, it is most effective when pinpointing images and building to a strong, even surprising last line.
Guidelines:

— As with acrostics, it is best to do a group tanka or cinquain on the tablet so that the students get the feel of counting syllables and sharpening images.

Examples:

Cherry memories —
Changing the appearance of
A street in springtime;
As we drive about we feel
Joyous and full of life, too!

— Emily Zerbe, BRNC

The misty mountains
Spring boldly out of the haze;
Sharp shapes cut the sky,
No longer melt into space,
But standing upright as one.

— Dorothy Yates, BRNC

Electric sound stabs,
Scarlet crashes into orange,
Marble chips pierce flesh,
Shakespeare shows us man's dark heart—
Nobody said art was safe!

—Carol F. Peck

b. Cinquain

I use two basic forms of the five-line cinquain:

Form 1: 2 syllables, 4 syllables, 6 syllables, 8 syllables, 2 syllables (no other restrictions).

Examples:

Forest
Wandering blind
One comes suddenly out
Into the sunlit world of day
Brightly

—Dorothy Yates, BRNC

The soul—
Continence of
All that bonds man ever
To his accountability
For life.

—Helen L. Anderson, BRNC

Water
Flowing swiftly
Sometimes a path or road
Now just a watery playground
River

—Joan Brindley, BRNC

Form 2:

— 1 noun to name your subject;
— 2 adjectives (or a 2-word metaphor) to describe it;
— 3 verbs to show what it does;
— 4 words that make a statement about it — maybe how it makes you feel;
— 1 word that is another word for it, a synonym.

Examples:

Trees
Sturdy, spreading
Entertain, nourish, surround
A place of beauty
Homes

         — Catherine J. Curtin, BRNC

God
Omnipresent, omnipotent
Creates, guides, heals
Made all spiritual reality
Life

         — Dorothy Emerson, BRNC

Grandchildren
Gene recognizable
Love, stimulate, remind
Extend life into eternity
Fulfillment

         — Helen L. Anderson, BRNC

 Occasionally I bring in an object to serve as the poem's subject, such as a lighted candle or a Chinese jade horse:

Light
Pure, steadfast
Shining, warming, illuminating

Spreading knowledge, bringing cheer
Hope

—Dorothy Yates, BRNC

Horse
Chinese art
Sitting, seeing, awakening
Looking back, ever powerful
Masterwork

—Anna Goldschmidt, BRNC

Horse
Graceful, suspicious
Jumping, seeking, finding
Searching for a friend
Hero

—Leila King, BRNC

3. Recipes

Nearly everyone in the group was thoroughly familiar with recipes for foods, but few had thought of using this approach to cooking with words. They seemed delighted by this unusual approach to poetry — enough familiar structure to make it easy to get started, yet enough freedom to let the imagination go and to bend the assignment somewhat. Some years I asked for a recipe for anything, and the range of results was wide — from how to raise cats or how to be a good bookkeeper to how to stay young at heart. Other times I focused it on a season, holiday, or idea. For the most part, they wrote with confidence and zest — once in a while someone would misunderstand and write an actual food recipe, but there is no harm in that.

Guidelines:

— You might start by asking how many of them like to cook and have favorite, foolproof recipes — but make it clear that you are not collecting real food recipes that day!
— Ask if they have ever thought of using the recipe format to write about ideas, feelings, or events.
— On the tablet write "Ingredients" and "Method" — the two essentials for any recipe. Point out that real recipes list specific amounts of each ingredient and that their recipes need specific amounts, too — write "List *specific* amounts" under "Ingredients." Under "Method," brainstorm with them for all the specific verbs they can think of that appear in recipes — "mix," "stir," "beat," "whip," "fold in," "combine," "knead," "roll out," "separate," etc.
— Specify a particular focus, if any, and summarize that they are to use the two-part recipe format for their poems, listing specific ingredients and describing how to put them together.

Examples:

RECIPE FOR SPRING

One half pound of hot sun
A jug full of rain
Handful of flowers
Pinch of leaves
A bowl full of egg sacs
A potful of praying mantises
1 pound of strawberries
3 jugs of narcissi
7 barrels of orange daffodils

Take one half pound of hot sun. Mix it with a jug of rain, a handful of flowers, a pinch of leaves, a bowl full of egg sacs. Pour all together and mix!

—Niya Bass, Grade 1

RECIPE FOR A PEACEFUL WORLD

3 cups peace
1/2 cup robots
4 cups rainbows
6 cups funniness
8 cups mothers

Put robots into the world to clean it and water the plants. Add rainbows all at once. Add funniness by getting clowns. Spread peace all around. Add mothers to take care of children. They will be peaceful because they do not have to clean.

—Conor Murphy, Grade 1

RECIPE FOR A PEACEFUL WORLD

50 cups of silence
10 cups of church
1/2 teaspoon of grumpiness
3 cups of rainbows to fill the sky with beauty
1 Tablespoon roses
5 cups clouds

Take the clouds and fill the sky up with them. Then take rainbows to make the sky beautiful. It's the beginning of the whole world being peaceful. Next take roses and plant around every cottage. Dig deep in the ground and bury the grumpiness. Go all the way to town and put churches in the most beautiful places in town. Put silence all over the world.

—Audrey Russek, Grade 1

RECIPE FOR HAPPINESS

Ingredients

A good heart
A happy look—rouge and a smile
Thoughts about happy things
Red poinsettias all around you
Happy feelings that take over your whole body

Method

Go into your heart to find the feelings. Mix the look with the thoughts and add. Surround yourself with the red poinsettias.

—Dorothy Oest, BRNC

RECIPE FOR SPRING

2 cups very small leaves, part green, part brown
1 Tablespoon small yellow flowers
Plenty of sunshine combined with
A little rain
Enough wind to blow *your* dandelion seeds into the next guy's
     yard
A cup of oil for the lawn mower and
1 quart of liniment for the back

—Joan Brindley, BRNC

RECIPE FOR SPRING

Ingredients

A world of people conversing and planning and anticipating
     clothes
9 million quarts of sunshine and fresh air
A garden
A new way of living

Method

Leave warmth and comfort of inside and take your problems to the fresh air and sunshine, then live and enjoy spring. It is later than you think. And do not feel you are a glutton if you take all day.

—Eleanor O'Brien, BRNC

THANKSGIVING DAY RECIPE

To make Thanksgiving Day a beautiful, perfect day from dawn to dusk, one needs very few ingredients—enveloped in the greatest of all envelopers.

On awakening give thanks for all blessings that come to mind. Take an attitude of praise—find something to praise—toward everyone you meet. Inwardly bless every person and every situation you encounter; outwardly, say, "Thank you!" for each bit of help from another. Thanking. Praising. Blessing.

Fold these, combine these components, enclose these in the greatest thing in the world, Love, and you will have all needed ingredients not just for a beautiful, perfect Thanksgiving Day but for every other day of your life.

—Vida Hickerson, BRNC

HALF A RECIPE FOR A LIFE TO BE THANKFUL FOR

Nature has provided us with a many-columned list of
Nourishing ingredients, exotic flavors, and food that creamily
Flow through our welcoming mouths,
But there are no directions for how to stir
Or where to measure how much,
And how do we weigh what we ought to know?
All of these things we learn too slowly
Or ponder, too long perhaps,
Hoping to finish the dish
Before the fire to cook it
Embers itself to an ash!

—Helen L. Anderson, BRNC

4. Borrowing Another Poet's Form

Occasionally a professional poet's poem strikes me as offering an excellent form for students to imitate. Such a poem is William Carlos Williams' widely anthologized "The Red Wheelbarrow," which has three vividly contrasting images and a provocative first line, "So much depends upon"—this focuses the images and turns them into a poem implying something about beauty, for one thing. By using the same first line but three different images, students can achieve a similarly tight poem, with unity, variety and progression all in four or five lines. Some may veer from the strict pattern, but somehow that focusing first line strengthens any approach and helps everyone get started.

Guidelines:

—Copy all but the first line of "The Red Wheelbarrow" onto the tablet—you are sharing with them a poem that isn't quite a poem, yet.
—Add the first line and ask how it changes the effect, what Williams is implying—answers will range from the purely practical—the farmer depends on the wheelbarrow to help in his work—to the aesthetic—the nature of beauty.
—Underline the first line and ask students to copy it onto their papers; then ask them to try to find three contrasting images that will somehow hang together when placed under that line.
—If people seem really stuck, suggest narrowing the focus to a time of day, a particular place, a season, an animal, etc.

Examples:

So much depends upon
Stars shining in the heavens,
Sounds of bells ringing,
And the gay Christmas tree.

—Betty Graham, BRNC

So much depends upon
The alligators at dusk,
The smell of the grass,
The feel of cool, smooth sheets.

—Betty Graham, BRNC

NOTE: This was a reworking of her earlier poem about summer—see Chapter I—some poets may want to try this is a tightening technique for earlier work.

So much depends upon
The bright sunny sky—
All nature is stimulated,
Forcing reluctant vegetation.

—Dorothy Yates, BRNC

So much depends upon
The lovely springtime,
The sound of bells
(Which you can never get enough of)
And being lucky enough to hear it!

—Dorothy Oest, BRNC

So much depends upon
When you say, "I do":
A life of joy or
A life of misery—
You will know after
A year is over.

—Anna Goldschmidt, BRNC

Another professional poem whose first line works well as a stim-ulator is "Pied Beauty," by Gerard Manley Hopkins. After that initial "Glory be to God for dappled things," he goes on to build a breathtaking array of vivid images to *show* their beauty. I ask stu-dents to use the same first line, substituting another adjective for "dappled," and likewise to build a convincing series of vivid im-ages.

Guidelines:

—Share "Pied Beauty" with the class, taking time to appreciate the imagery; it is such a packed poem that I read it twice.
—Mention how Hopkins makes a statement but then "proves" it through skillful use of many vivid specifics.
—Explain that the students will be borrowing his first line and overall structure, but that each will choose another adjective to replace "dappled."
—Brainstorm for suitable adjectives and write them on the tab-let—words like "shining," "glowing," "sparkling," "daz-zling," "fluffy," "shadowy," "glistening," "blooming," etc.
—Copy "Glory be to God for _____ things" on the tablet and remind them to be as specific as possible in their images.

Examples:

Glory be to God for glowing things . . .
For the sun which shines over you;
For the light that comes when you're good;
For the scary lightning dot that comes when you're bad;
For the glowing flowers that come in spring;
For all the glittering ocean that comes in the summer;
For the sparkling leaves that come in the fall;
For the white light snow that comes in winter;
And best of all, the light that comes when you learn.

—Antonia Fasanelli, Grade 4

Glory be to God for majestic things:
For castles, glorious with victory,
For deserts sandy and desolate,
And for black cats,
So strange and mysterious;
Glory be to God for pyramids
Flashing in the sun;
And best of all,
Glory be to God for
   Icicles
      melting in the moonlight.

—Nate Heller, Grade 3

Glory to God for things with the depth called black —
The crow, the grackle and the licorice stick,
The good dark dress and Negro man,
And the gaping emptiness, so holy high,
Undefined but by its awesome name.

—Helen L. Anderson, BRNC

Glory be to God for shining things —
Sunshine on flowers,
Moonlight on snow,

Diamonds in a necklace,
And people's eyes.

—*Sarah McInteer, BRNC*

Glory be to God for little things—
The tiny snowflake drifting toward the ground,
So different from all the others;
A single raindrop falls down but needs the
Assistance of friends to make a flower come to life;
A tiny baby, completely different from all the others—
It can grow up to be *anything*!
Who knows what it will be?
A small penny can mysteriously grow into
Thousands of dollars (That's what my mother said),
And where would whales be without plankton?

—*Joan Brindley, BRNC*

Glory be to God for stippled horses from sweat
Or stippled by color;
I was happy to ride a horse called White Marsh
When I was down in Anne Arundel County
During fairly warm days.
She was a hard horse to pull in
And once rode me between two trees and
Gave me a twisted shoulder;
I had to go to a doctor on the way back
To pull my shoulder into place.
I loved White Marsh—
Glory be to God for White Marsh!

—*Vanetta H. Bealle, BRNC*

Occasionally I have devoted two or three sessions to poems by
just one professional poet, such as Robert Frost, Emily Dickinson,
or William Carlos Williams and have drawn the writing ideas from
them. For example, when I read Frost's "The Road Not Taken"
and "Stopping by Woods on a Snowy Evening" the idea was one
of choices—what roads have you taken? Have you ever stopped to

consider or wondered about those *not* taken? Where might they
have led you?

Examples:

Stopping — a word and action not much used today;
Stop and look at the wonders here —
See the tiny flowers,
See the flight of a bird,
Watch the actions of our fellow humans;
All have purpose,
All follow a plan;
We see what has been done,
But what small parts escape us?
We miss the details and thus miss
A large part of life.

—Dorothy Yates, BRNC

THE ROAD NOT TAKEN

When I was a young girl
I had to choose between two roads —
To become a doctor or to get married.
I chose the second one, was never sorry to have done so.
It gave me two lovely children, six grandchildren,
And they are all the biggest pleasure of my life.
Though my marriage did not last too long,
I wonder what would have happened if I had chosen
    the other road?
Would I be happy today?
Maybe I would,
With the conviction to have been a help to many people.
Going back is impossible,
But I still did something
The other road would have led me to —
I chose to do some nursing when I was about 60 years old.
I had the benefit of both roads, that way,
But I never regretted my first choice.

—Anna Goldschmidt, BRNC

5. Opposites Attract — And Organize

Another framework that is not a form but which helps to organize a poem and get it started is the idea of playing opposites against each other — swift and slow, old and new, black and white, loud and soft, etc. Sometimes a student will choose to focus on just one half of the pair, which is fine — the opportunity is still there for variety and progression.

Guidelines:

- Read "Swift Things Are Beautiful" by Elizabeth Coatsworth (not in any anthologies in the Bibliography, but a children's librarian should be able to help you locate it). Dwell a bit on her vivid images and how some of the words even *sound* swift and slow. Point out how the contrasts strengthen the poem.
- Summarize the idea on the tablet: "Write a poem about swift and slow beauty — perhaps one stanza of swift and one of slow — or put the slow first — or alternating lines of swift and slow. Try for vivid images and sounds that will *show* the contrasts."
- If you offer other choices during this session, write them down too — old and new, black and white, etc. Maybe the class can think of more.

Examples:

SWIFT AND SLOW BEAUTY

Swift things are beautiful,
Like a star shooting from the sky,
Like a squirrel scattering up a tree,
Like a crab shooting down his hole,
Like water racing through the water faucet,
Like a fan going 'round and 'round.
Slow things are nice, too,
Like your heart going thump, thump,
Like a turtle walking out of the water,
Like the clouds moving in the sky,
Like a tomato turning red,
Like a clock going tick, tick, tick,
Like a kitten sneaking up on a bird,

Like the sunset going down,
Like your body growing.

—Elizabeth Kolsky, Grade 4

SWIFT AND SLOW

Swift is . . .
My hand reaching for a plum,
Running in a nice, cool breeze,
A squirrel running up a tree,
The wind running in the sky,
An icy cold brook taking its jog.
Slow is . . .
A snowflake walking to the ground,
Putting spinach where it's supposed to go,
A cloud walking to the other end,
A sunset getting its colors.

—Laurie Bowles, Grade 4

Swift is a pelican diving and catching that fish;
Swift is also a mouse escaping that cat;
Slow is the tide gradually coming in —
You're not aware of anything,
But suddenly your feet are wet!
Slow is also how the time seems to go
As a child sits in school
And waits for vacation to begin.

—Joan Brindley, BRNC

SLOW THINGS ARE BEAUTIFUL

The opening of a rosebud,
The attempts of a young bird to fly,
The first steps of a child,
The building of a cathedral —
These things give the viewer
Time to observe the beauty
Within each growing object,
Increasing in beauty
As time slowly passes.

—Dorothy Yates, BRNC

Swift things are beautiful —
An airplane wobbling in the air,
Sounding very noisy —
A horse running free in a meadow,
My thoughts when I'm remembering horses.

—Betty Graham, BRNC

D. REMEMBERING THE PAST

Life is a patchwork quilt
Held together by the threads of memory —
A song recalls a person, a place,
A dance, a parade, a concert —
The notes of a song
Pull the threads of life
From the dim past
Toward the light of today.

—Dorothy Yates, BRNC

Older people have much knowledge, expertise and just plain experience that can add richly to their poems, but they do not necessarily think of the past poetically. All it takes is a little suggesting, a little focusing, on the part of the workshop leader, and some wonderful memories come forth.

1. Traces of Our Roots

Young and old alike are fascinated by their roots, and one of my favorite writing ideas is to have people consider their roots and write about the traces of those, especially the places, that are still evident in themselves.
Guidelines:

— Introduce the idea by talking about roots — people will be interested in sharing information about their own family roots.
— Move on to the idea of looking for traces of our roots still evident in us — characteristics of the country or its people that we still have, even if we have to stretch our imaginations a bit.
— Summarize the writing project on the tablet: "Write a poem

about your roots, showing the specific traces that still show in you.''

Examples:

ROOTS

The stuff in me is
The sand of the Sinai Desert;
Moses' cane is my backbone;
The Red Sea is my blood;
All those things are in me—
I am in them, too.

—Noah Bickart, Grade 3

AFRICA

My hair is the color of ebony;
My eyes are the color of a log;
My skin is the color of the soil;
My hands are as soft as a rabbit's skin;
My legs are like leopards' legs,
And I have the kindness of a deer;
My eyebrows are like grassy hills;
My eyelashes are as long as the day;
My clothes are as brown as the dirt;
My feet are as little as a stone;
I have the brain of an owl,
And I'm as strong as a king;
I sleep so quiet, like a lamb,
I am as sensitive as a squirrel;
My fingers move along the piano
As a coyote moves across the prairie;
I am as bright as the sun,
And I love the delicious foods,
For I am from Africa.

—Dawn Dew, Grade 3

THE TRAVELER

I am a traveler.
In German,
     Reisner means traveler.
My ancestors were travelers.
 I travel in
        Planes,
           Boats,
              Cars
                 and in
     my imagination too.
In my imagination
     I travel
         to
     other worlds,
       other galaxies,
   other universes and
   new adventures.
I travel past
        black holes,
    quasars,
          supernovas,
exploding galaxies and
             sometimes
I pass
   Betelgeuse.

                      —Josh Reisner, Grade 3

My father was once facing a difficult time in his life—
He was a school teacher, a school principal;
I noticed as a young girl that he sought solace
In purchasing an old printing press and spending
Many hours in libraries looking into our family's roots,
Writing them down in conversational style
And printing copies for his three children—
I should see if my copy is still hiding among my papers.
We are traced back to English forbears on one side

And to Admiral Dewey on the other side;
I remember one interesting point—
My sisters and I are closely related to John Alden and his wife
    Priscilla;
That may account for my interest in young people's love affairs!
England brings me my love for reading, writing and teaching;
Today brings my interest back to Dad's printed story of our
    heritage—
I must look it up.

—Dorothy Emerson, BRNC

I am wonderfully American,
My line long settled here;
I married a man nearer to his Swedish roots
And I bore three children
With great long bones and tawny hair,
And we throve on pancakes, herring and dark bread;
We loved good cheese
And celebrated Christmas the eve before.
But the color green speaks life to me—
I love misty skies
And the anger of the sea,
I laugh loud and talk too much
But with quiet in my voice,
And I hear music in a thousand ways
That others never know;
I love potatoes
And my whiskey straight
And my maiden name was Kelly.

—Helen L. Anderson, BRNC

Variation: Grandparents

Guidelines:

—Ask students to write about some less remote ancestors—their
    grandparents.

- —Summarize on the tablet: "What did they look like? Sound like? Smell and feel like? Make you feel? What did they do with you? What other special things do you remember about them?"
- —Remind students to be as specific as possible.

Examples:

Grandmother has the dust of nature's hand on her body. She has the frost spread across her once-brown hair. She's the warmth of fire. She is beautiful as a silvery cool river rushing against the shore. She is lovable as sunlight on a running river. She is warm as fur. She is the first one up and the last to bed. When she is sad I share her grief with sorrow. Her face is rosy scarlet, shining green eyes, and silver streams of hair. She makes the bread which honey is spread on in the morning. At lunch time she makes a casserole with peas, beef, lima beans, broccoli, carrots with bread and ham. Next she serves *tocino morcilla* and something else I can't remember. Anyway, for lunch we drink milk which was milked that morning from the cows. And at supper we eat meat or noodles and for dessert, pie.

—*Julio Corrales, Grade 4*

BOPPA

I have a grandfather—his special name is Boppa;
Boppa is a hard-working retired football coach;
Boppa is a gardener, always pulling weeds;
Boppa is a sightseer, always going to Europe with Gramma;
Boppa is a true fisherman, fishing from his dock;
Boppa is always tan from swimming or walking along the beach;
Boppa is always having me on his lap, insisting I don't grow up,
　　flashing a wonderful smile, twinkling his eyes at me,
Loving me always.

—*Stephanie Blackman, Grade 4*

I don't think of my two grandmothers' hair as gray—
I think of it as silver;
My mom's mom's skin is wrinkled,
But I just think it's smiling;
My dad's mom has veiny hands,

But *I* know it's not oldness,
It's a sign of higher intelligence.
My grandfather isn't bald,
It's just that his scalp needs
A breath of fresh air;
My grandfather laughs at my dumb jokes
And makes me feel special.

—Jennifer Stewart, Grade 4

SUPER PLUMP AND JUICY GRANDPARENTS!

Grandparents are
            MYSTERIOUS
With hair
                that seems to
        Glow
        in the
        Dark
Grandparents remind
me of
        ESCARGOT
when they move
They give me a balanced
    meal without
            vegetables
They take you to
                horror movies
EVEN though they
don't like them, so
        BOO!
My grandma is like a flower
My grandpa is like grass
because they always take
care of you.
Super Plump and Juicy
Grandparents are
BEAUTIFUL! and
pull your cheeks!

—Julian Turner, Grade 4

My grandmother had grey eyes;
Her hair was snow white and wavy;
She had love enough to spread over her many
    children and grandchildren;
She told us vivid stories of her life in pre
    and Civil War Virginia;
Her understanding and sympathy,
Her wit and sense of humor
Endeared her to young and old;
Her memory is a source of
Knowledge and love
To all who knew her.

                —Dorothy Yates, BRNC

My paternal grandfather was a retired minister
    and was fond of children;
He had a small farm with a few cows;
We loved to go there because he gave us such a good time:
We could jump in the hay mows, drive the horses,
    and sing around the piano—one of his daughters could play;
He had a reddish beard and I thought he was old,
But he died at about sixty, so he could not have been old;
Both of my grandmothers were second wives and
I don't remember much about them.

                —Emily Zerbe, BRNC

"Grandparents" is a strange subject to me—
I never really remember any grandparents.
Children say to me, "You remind me of my grandmother";
I think they mean I am lively;
I never think of myself as a grandparent;
I couldn't really be one anyway
Because I never married,
And being only 92, almost 93,
I haven't stopped being a child yet.

                —Dorothy Emerson, BRNC

2. Childhood Favorites

Everyone has a wealth of childhood memories that can be tapped into. I have found it best to focus the writing assignment on one particular childhood favorite at a time, such as a place, a toy, foods, a teacher, etc.

Guidelines:

— This idea is easy to introduce in informal conversation with the group — people can usually remember at least one favorite right away, and one person's memory stimulates another person's. The examples help, too.
— Remind people to be as specific as possible in their details:
— For places, write on the tablet, "What was your favorite or secret place? When did you go there? What did it look, sound, smell and feel like? Did you ever take anybody else there?"
— For a favorite toy, "Who gave it to you? What did it look, sound, and feel like? What did you like best about it? What ever happened to it?"
— For favorite foods, "Who made them for you? What made them special? How did they taste, smell, look and feel?"
— For a favorite teacher, " What did he or she teach? Where and when? What did he or she look like? Dress like? Sound like? What made him or her special to you? What did you learn from him or her besides the subject?" NOTE: There is a wonderful example poem by Lenore Coberly on pp. 84-85 of *Writers Have No Age*, "Olaf Hougen was Eighty-five Last Night."

Examples:

FAVORITE PLACE

I spent the summers in Michigan
On the shores of Eagle Lake
Near a dairy farm —
Fresh milk every day for us kids,
Cool, rich and creamy —
Blossoming trees —
Skunks used to come and drive us crazy!
In the evening we used to have a special gathering

And walk to Paw Paw—right by Mother's house—
And go to the movies.
There were two horses who pulled a carriage
With room for six or seven people—
We'd ride into Lawton.
We used to get hungry
And eat the grapes next door.

—*Betty Graham, BRNC*

FAVORITE TOY

My favorite toy when I was very small?
My teddy bear!
He was quite large,
A real armful.
I loved him to death—
Till his arms got limp and his fur got thin.
I finally gave him up when
I was given a beautiful doll with real hair
And for whom I loved to make clothes—
What a wardrobe she had!
Poor teddy, fickle me.

—*Alice Kennedy, BRNC*

I had a doll about three or four feet long
And she had a beautiful head of hair;
It came off, one day—
I didn't mean to take it off—
And I saw the inside of her head—
Her eyes were blinking and blinking—
It spoiled her for me to see them;
She had beautiful eyes.
She had pretty shoes and her arms bent;
Her legs bent at the knees and ankles.
She was like a living doll—
She was real to me.
I loved her terribly—
No matter where I was,
If I had that doll in my lap

I was happy.
I wish I still had her!

—Marjorie Monroe, BRNC

She was my dearest toy—
Four inches tall and just ten cents.
I know, because I bought her
With money to spend on vacation fun.
She was made of stone and elastically jointed;
Her wig was thumbnail small and often slid awry;
Yellow crayon carefully applied to the hole-centered skull
Provided better indication.
Her shoes were painted on
And she was very sensibly named Helen!
She lived in bureau drawers,
Retired buffet cabinets, cozy closets,
And even once a doll house.
She had many clothes and we talked a lot.
She went with me on my wedding night
And then no longer mattered.
The last time I saw her she was a sorry sight,
And all the memories were long snuffed out
With pictures of round fat babies
With demanding flesh and lovely eyes
Of doting recognition,
All of whom were growing up
And never could be purchased.

—Helen L. Anderson, BRNC

FAVORITE FOODS

When there was a special day and there was a pie
The extra crust was the best part of all—
Rolled out very thin and spread with melted butter,
Sprinkled with brown sugar and cinnamon,
Then made into a long tube and cut into many slices,
Placed then on a cookie pan,
Put in a very hot oven for a minute or two,

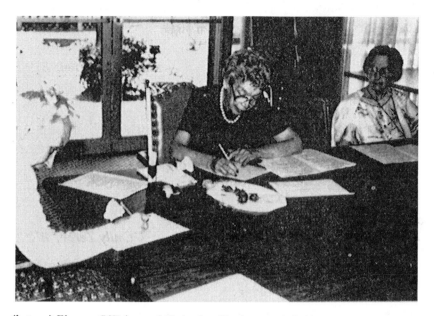

(l. to r.) Eleanor O'Brien and Catherine Curtin start their "strawberry" poems as Dona Clapp reads poems written the previous week.
Photo by Wendy C. Webster.

And someone says, "These are for you" —
Oh, those wonderful "stickies"
One never forgets.

— Marie Huff, BRNC

My memory always takes me back to delicious
Homemade bread and the time consumed in achieving
Fourteen loaves and two tins of biscuits for a family each week.
We started the night before and each took turns
Cranking the old bread mixer;
Then my mother started early next morning,
Rolling, kneading and baking;
Everyone liked my mother's homemade bread,
Especially the kids across the street,
And we loved their "store boughten" bread;

Instead of fancy confections or cakes,
The "special" every day was brown sugar
On plain homemade bread.

—Eleanor O'Brien, BRNC

My favorite food? Peaches—
We did not live in peach country,
But they were shipped in, in bushel baskets.
First we ate the ripe ones and then
At canning time we ate the poor ones or parts.
They were so good on ice cream or
Served with sugar and cream.
Peaches are a sweet memory.

—Emily Zerbe, BRNC

FUDGE

Gooey, chewy, yummy fudge,
A dark brown river
Flowing over a patch of snow
And leaving a little dark brown pool
In the bottom of the container.
The taste of that dark brown pool
Had to last till you got the next
Gooey, chewy, yummy fudge!

—Joan Brindley, BRNC

SUCCULENT MEMORIES

With a few hoarded pennies one could
Spend lavishly in the town dry goods store—
Horehound sticks and licorice balls
Were favorite purchases,
Also candy hearts with verses in red;
At home, quince honey on hot biscuits
Or strawberry preserves cooked in the sun
Made a delicious supper treat;
Taffy pulls, resulting in blisters on fingers
Furnished entertainment for children's parties;
Childhood appetites were fresh and keen,

With strong likes and dislikes;
Age often jades the sense of taste.

—Dorothy Yates, BRNC

FAVORITE TEACHERS

Memorable teacher?
Could there be such a creature?
And was the subject math?
Strange to say, that was the path
The teacher took me —
Little stories and anecdotes,
Mixed with plain, old fashioned $6+3=9$
Made her a memorable teacher,
One I'll never forget.

—Alice Kennedy, BRNC

Professor Bugbee taught Ancient History in eighth grade, and *he* was ancient, as far as I was concerned. He had reddish gray hair and his suits were always wrinkled. He never was dressed properly, and I think that means a lot. His handkerchief was always half hanging out of his pocket (I told him about it one day and he didn't take kindly to it — gave me two demerits, which campused me, since I already had eight). He sounded kind of sissified but was an excellent teacher.

He was a very kind person — I think I learned to be kind from him. I was in Detention Study and he was kind when I was in there — he'd say, "Let's go over tomorrow's study program," and he did help me a lot. The day of Class Day he wrote: "In the 16th century it was Romeo and Juliet,/Today it is Richards and Balliet" and gave me two dolls representing Luther and me. By the time I graduated, he was one of my very best friends.

—Alice Balliet, BRNC

Teachers are a cup of tea —
I learned from him what is patience;
Sometimes I was a flat tire without him.
Like tea, teachers lift your spirits.

—Catherine J. Curtin, BRNC

3. The Good Old Days

There are many ways to look back over several decades, share memories, and write about the past. The focusing ideas that have worked best with my group fall into four categories: (a) remembering how various things used to be; (b) remembering a specific age; (c) things we wish we had said or done; and (d) inventions and discoveries that have changed the world.

Guidelines:

— (a) For a topic as broad as "Remember When," I have found it best to list on the tablet several categories the writers might like to consider, such as fashions, hair styles, transportation, machines, entertainment, social activities, employment, and any others they may suggest. And one time I read them *Momilies* and asked them to write about things their mothers always said to them or warned them about.

Examples:

REMEMBER WHEN . . .

I remember going to the A&P grocery every Saturday
And buying a lot of sugar and flour, lard, a bag of potatoes
And cream cake;
The store always smelled like coffee;
It had a wooden floor
And the people wore white aprons —
They were young village people and were very sociable.

—Alice Caton, BRNC

I remember . . .
Wearing short dresses above the knee;
Rumble seats in cars — kids would all pile in,
    the more the merrier;
Long manes of hair;
Vaudeville — my brother loved the theater
    and would drag me along —
I loved vaudeville and it was good —

he was very particular about what he saw;
The Bunny Hop, the Charleston;
Foods—well, when we were in school,
    we just loved to eat anything around—
    that doesn't change—
My mother always had something baked!

                    —Lottie Bennett, BRNC

DO YOU REMEMBER . . .
Garter belts?
On machines, we had lawnmowers you had to push—
    all lawns seemed to be uphill;
Remember those huge bouffant hair styles?
Almost everyone teased their hair and
Some wore what were called Beehives—
Some looked just right for a bird to build its nest in;
I still remember vaudeville—
I didn't know it was going out,
So I sat and laughed at George Burns, Jack Benny, and Will
    Rogers,
And there were many others, too;
When a boy took me dancing, we danced cheek to cheek—
Today's dancers look as if they don't even know each other;
I have to mention one other thing—
What became of the penny postcard?

                    —Joan Brindley, BRNC

DO YOU REMEMBER . . .

Fishtail coats that the ladies wore back in the 30's? The expectant mothers liked them especially, because they were full in the back which made it nobody's business if your stomach was getting larger and larger;

Spanish shawls, which were very beautiful and popular back in the twenties? But we could never even consider such frivolous and expensive items—they were just for people with money, but you saw lots of them in all different pretty colors;

High shoes that laced up above your ankles? Whenever we wanted new shoes, my mother would tell us that we would have to

be careful; we wore them out too fast—when she was a child, she had to wear brass-topped shoes so they would not wear out so fast;
Veils on hats to cover the face and for style?

The first permanent wave machines that used to scare you just to look at them? And whenever you got a wave, everyone in town came to see the new miracle machine that, like Halley's Comet, they might never see again;
Minstrel shows presented by local talent?

—Eleanor O'Brien, BRNC

MOMILIES

"I can't get you up and I can't get you to bed";
"Choose your friends carefully";
"Be friendly to everyone but intimate with few";
"Don't talk about the things you hear at home";
"Don't waste your time and eyesight reading trash";
"Eat at least a little of everything on your plate."

—Dorothy Yates, BRNC

"Don't eat seafood or you'll get ill";
"Don't mix seafood with sweet stuff";
"Behave yourself in public";
"Don't associate with people who have poor manners";
"A lady doesn't cross her legs so her petticoat shows—
    she crosses her feet nicely";
"He hasn't been brought up like you have";
"Be home on time";
"You can stay and talk with so-and-so but don't make it long";
"If you kiss him, you'll have a fever like he has."

—Vanetta Bealle, BRNC

How proudly sits my daughter
    with her daughter in her arms;
Her ways are fresher, her systems
    yet to be discovered;
But I know how often, when the need comes forth,
    she'll hear my voice
        re-echoed in her pseudo-stern admonishing,

Just as I heard my mother's
  and she must have heard hers,
As we each in turn pressed our young
To grow up with all the wonderful, old-fashioned virtues
  that made us as nice as I think we've been;
Yes, mama, I recall —
"Pride goeth before a fall."

— Helen L. Anderson, BRNC

— (b) in one of her poems, a class member had referred to A. E. Housman's poem "When I Was One-and-Twenty," and I thought that an excellent specific time for everyone to write about. After reading the Housman poem I asked everyone to use his title and write about being that age. On the tablet I wrote some leading questions: "What was going on in the world? What was going on in your life? Would you like to be 21 again? If so, why? If not, why not? Would you do anything differently?"

Examples:

WHEN I WAS ONE-AND-TWENTY

When I was twenty-one, I had graduated from high school and taken a short business course. I was looking for my place in the world, but like everyone else, I was overwhelmed by the Depression and depressed to the point no one would want me for a job or for a wife. No, I don't want to be twenty-one again. Even old age and sickness leave you with hope that things will be better, and you know that if you leave things to God, conditions will be better.

— Eleanor O'Brien, BRNC

When I was twenty-one, I was allowed to register to vote — I was tickled to death, because I had been working in a courthouse for a long time before that. Hoover was President, so the first time I voted I didn't have much of a choice, because Roosevelt was running. I became very active in Young Republicans.

I was unmarried, and my social life couldn't have been better. Dances were the most popular entertainment. I was also a joiner of any club I could get into. My big interest was politics and still is.

I'd love to be twenty-one again—I'd be back in Pennsylvania and I'd get right back into politics. I would not do a thing differently, except maybe I would have gotten married sooner. I've had a good life and no regrets!

—Alice Balliet, BRNC

When I was one-and-twenty,
Oh, so long ago,
When I was one-and-twenty,
There was much I didn't know;
Everything was lovely,
Everything serene;
Now I'm five and eighty
And view the years between.

—Alice Kennedy, BRNC

—(c) Ideas in this category included secret childhood desires, things we wish we had done or maybe not done, things we wish we had asked someone else—an idea from *Write Age* magazine—and things we wish we had written—an idea sparked by Alan Paton's essay in *Time*, April 25, 1988, in which he discussed things he would have been proud to have written. The leading question was simple: "What do you wish you had done, or asked, or written, and why?" This project could of course be stretched into three separate assignments.

Examples:

LOOKING BACK . . .

I would have loved to be a research scientist—
That is something you could give to the whole world;
They are learning all the time
And in learning are trying to achieve;
I would love to have gone to places I heard and read about,
Especially London in the spring, then Paris;
I wish I had known some of the great people in the world,
    such as both the Roosevelts—
I *did* once see Mrs. Roosevelt when she was invited to speak

To a gathering at a large hotel;
The security were pushing us aside,
And Mrs. Roosevelt was coming out with Mrs. Morgenthau —
I thought she was *beautiful*, a beauty from within.

— Lottie Bennett, BRNC

SECRET DESIRE

I would like to have known Bing Crosby
And to have heard my voice singing
"I'm dreaming of a white Christmas."

— Catherine J. Curtin, BRNC

I WISH I HAD ASKED

I could have asked my mother many things,
But I'm not sure she would have known the answer.
Today, with science and today's technology,
I know there is an answer.
Some things I'd like to know are —
Why are bubbles always round?
Why do stars seem to twinkle?
Why does the sea look blue?
I used to ask where do babies come from;
Today I know it had nothing to do with the stork.

— Joan Brindley, BRNC

I wish I had written the novels of Charles Dickens. The story developed in each novel is captivating and holds one's interest until the end. His understanding of human nature is great and his sense of humor delightful. I have enjoyed his writing since childhood and have re-read them often. They never cease to keep my interest.

— Dorothy Yates, BRNC

— (d) This idea was quite self-focusing — the class wrote about significant inventions within their lifetimes and how they have changed the world. One time I limited them to the single most important invention or discovery *ever* and its effect on the world.

Examples:

SIGNIFICANT INVENTIONS

The man on the moon —
I don't know how he got there!
It makes me feel I could do it,
But I don't dare!
The victrola — I used to like to play it,
Benny Goodman, especially;
I heard people sing on it — one was Frank Sinatra;
Television — I'm glad it was invented,
But sometimes I get awfully tired of it!

— Vanetta Bealle, BRNC

What invention could the world not possibly do without?
The wheel is necessary to the modern world
    as it was to the ancient;
It is true that the Inca, the Mayan, the Egyptian
Built their marvelous structures without the wheel,
But they had unlimited slave power held in subjection;
The wheel freed man from domination of forced labor
And let him develop his mind and soul with great ideas.

— Dorothy Yates, BRNC

The one discovery the world could not possibly do without is electricity. It gives us light and energy and makes our reading possible. Our food processing is done by electricity. Communication is faster and more widespread because of it, and we have a broader scope on life with it — through telephone and television. Our working facilities are greater now than they ever have been — typewriters in offices use electricity, our clothing is made with the help of electricity, the shoemaker could not fix our shoes without it, operating rooms depend on it, and we know the next president through electronics. All in all, it makes for a better life.

— Alice Balliet, BRNC

I THINK

The world could not possibly exist
Without the ability to think—
Everything begins with thought;
We see and hear mentally first,
Then things come to life.

—*Dorothy Emerson, BRNC*

5. Encounters With Animals

Even if people never had pets, most have had at least one meaningful experience with an animal in the past. This assignment asks
the writer to describe that encounter so vividly that the reader feels
the impact, knows how the writer felt about it.
Guidelines:

- There are several superb professional poems that will show
  students what you mean by vivid description of a meaningful
  encounter: "A Narrow Fellow in the Grass" by Emily Dickinson; "The Darkling Thrush" by Thomas Hardy; "The Tyger"
  by William Blake; and "The Fish" by Elizabeth Bishop.
- On the tablet write the framework: "*Encounter With An Animal.* Describe what happened in detail—what was the animal?
  Describe its look, sound, smell, texture, and especially movements. Show how you felt."

Examples:

CATERPILLAR

All humped upon the twig you gripped,
You jerked in rhythm as you slipped
Your final skin, then silently
Became a hard shell fastened by
Two filaments of steely lace.
We put you in a glassy place,
And still as stone you sheltered there,
Of sun and starlight unaware;

But some primordial pulse beat on
And brought you to a breathless dawn.

—Carol F. Peck

OPOSSUM

With startling introduction
    We met our opossum
Peering through a window,
    Clinging almost desperately
To an ice-glazed shrub
    On a cold-stilled day.
He wintered well on our side porch
    With lush fruit
And whatever suited his unknown fancy
    That we tried always to discover.
He snuggled warmly in a quilt
    That had often known
Small human forms and
    Once or twice a cat.
And then came a February day
    All garnished with promises of spring,
And our possum withdrew his
    Silent needs for human recognition
And desperately bloodied his
    Thin clawed paws
In his struggle to get free.
We unlatched the door and
    Let him go,
Leaving small red tracks
    In the melting snow,
And somehow saw eternity!

—Helen L. Anderson, BRNC

E. LOOKING TO THE FUTURE

Sometimes it is just as important to look forward as to remember the past. Our writing topics in this category have included reincarnation, filling a time capsule, being in charge of the world, predictions, and our own personal timelessness — our grandchildren.

1. Reincarnation As An Animal

As soon as I read Fleur Cowles *If I Were An Animal*, in which she gives the responses of more than one hundred celebrities who answer the question, "What would you choose to be if you could be reincarnated as an animal?" I knew the poetry group would love it. We all enjoyed many of the celebrity answers before the group answered the questions themselves.

Guidelines:

— You might have the group help decide which celebrity answers to read aloud — they may have favorite stars.
— Write the question on the tablet, adding, "Be sure to tell *why*. You might describe how you'd look and what you'd do all day and how you'd feel."

Examples:

If I were reincarnated
I'd like to come back as a
Pampered dog. Why?
I'd never have to cook;
When I got hungry
There would be food in my dish.
I'd never have to shop, either —
My owner would buy my collar and leash.
And I'd never ever have to worry about thieves —
I'd bury my treasures in the back yard,
Keeping an eye out for cats.
True, I'd have to suffer through a flea bath
Once in a while,

But this isn't so bad
If you remember to keep your eyes shut!

—Joan Brindley, BRNC

I'd come back as a skunk because nobody would ever bother or antagonize me. I'd be a loner and live in the country someplace, and at night I'd explore and look for food, because nobody is ever going to feed a skunk! Skunks relate to politics, too, because there are a lot of them in it!

—Alice Balliet, BRNC

If I were reincarnated I would not like to be an animal. They are at too much of a disadvantage as compared with man. Man can speak, write music, invent things, but animals would be very limited. Their life span would be limited, also. Animals are taken advantage of by man.

—Mrs. Zurawski, BRNC

2. Filling A Time Capsule

Writers of all ages like to imagine that they are in charge of deciding just what from our present world should go into a time capsule to be opened, perhaps centuries from now, by a future civilization.
   Guidelines:

- *After presenting the idea, talk with the group a bit about the representative specific*, single items that stand for certain aspects of our culture, such as particular books, pictures and music—ask them for some examples.
- On the tablet list some suggested categories: outdoor things, indoor things, things to see, hear, smell, taste, and touch, things that record ideas, etc.
- Stress that this is a poem—total, objective representation of our world is not the object so much as personal choices that will show what each poet feels is important and precious enough to be shown to future civilizations. Each capsule *should* be different.

—Stress variety of objects, too, and suggest that they even put in
some intangibles, if they like.

Examples:

If I had a time capsule
I would put the art of poetry in,
Some fresh snow,
The love of Mom;
I would put six pine needles in
And the freeness of our country;
I would put some wind in
And my favorite game;
I would put a school in
And a very pretty shell;
I would put a Martin Luther King speech in;
I would put a book in
And the happiness of Christmas;
I would put the coolness of water in
And a yummy pear.

—Joshua Goren, Grade 3

If I were to put some of my goals into a time capsule
I would choose some sculptures by Rodin;
I would also put in some paintings by Rembrandt;
I would put in my two gerbils;
I would put the Gettysburg Address by Abraham Lincoln in;
I would also put in the love of my family;
I would put in my favorite book, the *Guiness Book of World
      Records*;
I also would put in my AM/FM radio;
I would put the Bible in the time capsule;
One more thing—the world globe.

—Thaddeus Rudd, Grade 3

How should our world from the beginning
Be best represented for times to come?
Let us start with the Scriptures,

Then Shakespeare,
And the music of Beethoven,
The paintings of Rembrandt,
The voice of Caruso,
The ballet of Isadora Duncan,
And the political theories of Jefferson.

—Dorothy Yates, BRNC

Variation: Limit the contents to one sense, such as sounds.

SOUNDS FOR A TIME CAPSULE

I would recommend the sound of Niagara or Victoria Falls,
Have a survey of the people for their favorite music,
Sounds of an old-fashioned steam engine,
Sounds of a factory in full production,
The pleasant sound of a rambling stream of water through
the countryside
    which invites people to sit near it and have a picnic.

—Eleanor O'Brien, BRNC

The call of my mother to come in to my meals and do my chores;
The sound of the school bell ringing for *no* school that day;
Caruso singing in the opera house;
The sounds of all kinds of birds, except the blackbird;
The wind blowing through trees;
The whole sound of an automobile!

—Mrs. Edwards, BRNC

3. Wish Fulfillment

Projects in this category ranged from (a) being in charge of the world to (b) imagining a magic day.
Guidelines:

—(a) Read aloud Judith Viorst's delightful children's book, *If I Were In Charge of the World*. Tell the group that they, too, will be ruling the world in their poems—they can be silly or serious or, ideally, a mixture of the two. On the tablet write:

"What would you make legal and illegal? Think of both large and small issues, from world peace to what foods could be served." In a Presidential election year, we also did "If I Were President."

Examples:

IF I RULED THE WORLD

If I ruled the world
I would banish war
And settle all disagreements
By discussion and vote.
Justice would be the guideline —
All humans would have equal rights
Which must be constantly defended
Against the forces of evil.
This utopia is our dream;
May we never awaken to reality.

— *Dorothy Yates, BRNC*

If I ruled the world
I'd make widows who lost their husbands
And children who lost their fathers,
And had no one to support them,
Have no worries.
The widows would have no worries about food
And children would have no worries about shoes —
I'd see that they had food and shoes.

— *Lewis Blumenthal, BRNC*

If I were in charge of the world there would be no oatmeal;
There would be more trains in every direction;
There would be kites flying high for the pleasure of children;
There would be more country and only a few big towns;
There would be a theater in every town;
There would be many more libraries;
There would be no ten school years — eight should do;
There would be airplanes going to the moon;

There would be no military, no air force, but plenty of ships for a
  navy;
There would be a cooking stove in every home;
There would be lots of parks where animals could run around;
Everybody would have to marry and have two children,
to keep the amount of people up.

—Anna Goldschmidt, BRNC

IF I WERE PRESIDENT

I'd think how lucky I was to be President—
I'd have the biggest job in the country—
No one could take it away from me!
I'd like having all those servants
And living in the White House;
I'd even like making all those decisions;
That would make me proud—
Wouldn't it make you proud?

—Dorothy Oest, BRNC

—(b) Tell the class you are giving them a magic day—they can
   go anywhere, see anything, do anything, eat anything, meet
   anyone—ask them to be as specific as possible with sensory
   imagery, so that the reader will be able to have the same
   experience. Repeat the specifics on the tablet: "Where
   would you go? Why? What would you see? Do? Eat? Would
   you take anyone with you or meet anyone there?"

Examples:

ONE MAGIC DAY

For one magic day I would like to return
To the land of the rising sun
To a very special little street
With its many small shops so nice and neat,
Where you stroll along at a leisurely pace
And all shop owners greet you with a bow and smiling face;
You do not always need to buy,

It's just great that you stopped by;
The first place is the jewelry store
With the jade and pearl and much more,
The beautiful fabrics of cotton and silk,
The little store with the meat and milk,
Then the trimming place with buttons and lace
And many designs I would like to trace;
The little children with their almond eyes
Say, "Hi, Baby" and note your surprise!
Most of all the porcelain shop oh, so fine,
Makes you stop for a long, long time.
Gee, it's time to go home,
Again tomorrow I will roam.

—*Marie Huff, BRNC*

For just one day I'd like to run in
And see people I used to know in Pennsylvania
And to see Snigger, my dog, again—
I always wanted him with me!

—*Helen Shoemaker, BRNC*

For just one day I would like to fly to the North Pole;
For just one day I would like to be the President of the U.S.A.;
For just one day I would like to eat only potato soup;
For just one day I would like to visit Israel;
For just one day I would like to be the Queen of England;
For just one day I would like to see the world from outer space;
For just one day I would like to leave Washington, D.C.;
For just one day I would like to go to Switzerland, to try to climb
	the Jungfrau and look down from up there;
For just one day I would like to eat only ice cream.

—*Anna Goldschmidt, BRNC*

For just one day
I'd like longer than the usual twenty-four hours;
My Magic Day would give me time
To visit all the countries of the world
To compare cultures, religions, climates and topography,

To learn how and why peoples differ;
Knowledge promotes understanding,
Understanding promotes sympathy,
And sympathy leads to love and peace
Between peoples everywhere.

—Dorothy Yates, BRNC

Variation: Limit the idea to spending a day with a famous person each writer has always wanted to meet—"Whom would you choose? Why? Where would you go? What would you do together? What would you ask him or her?"

Examples:

ONE DAY WITH . . .

The person I would spend the day with is my mother—
I'd sit with her and talk about everything
And joke and share what we had been doing;
We'd go out to lunch at a restaurant;
She was great company,
But all my family were great company!

—Catherine J. Curtin, BRNC

A DAY WITH SHAKESPEARE

"Good morning, Mr. Shakespeare! Please tell me if you and you alone wrote everything attributed to you. It doesn't seem possible, but no one has ever been able to prove otherwise, although a number of people have been suggested.

"To whom were the sonnets addressed? Who was the lady of the sonnets? Was it Eve, as implied in your first line, or a contemporary of yours?

"Did you ever dream that over 2,000 quotations would be culled from your 37 plays and 154 sonnets?

"Are you aware of your lack of modesty when you said your words would outlast stone and steel and guarantee immortality to anyone you chose to write about?

"How could you have known so much philosophy? After all, you lived only 52 years.

"Did you think how you would be the forerunner of a principle of modern psychology and modern medicine when you wrote, 'A merry heart goes all the way; your sad tires in a mile.'

"Did you realize how many people in the future you would speak for when you wrote, 'My library was dukedom enough'?"

These questions, their answers, and a discussion of same would consume a day's time at least.

—Vida Hickerson, BRNC

4. Hopes and Predictions

January traditionally has us looking ahead and making resolutions for the new year. Instead I have had my class write their hopes or predictions either for the year ahead or the future in general.

Guidelines:

—Sometimes I leave the idea wide open; other times I write a framework on the tablet: "What are your hopes for the world? For the country? For the nursing home? For your family? For yourself?" which moves from the broad to the personal and could just as well be reversed, moving from the personal out to the broad.

—For predictions, I sometimes write some categories on the tablet, areas they may wish to consider, such as politics, world history, sports, fashion, hair styles, transportation, music, medicine, science, machines, food, famous people, etc.

Examples:

HOPES FOR 1987

I have such hopes for the coming year —
A lot of them I know aren't possible,
But I hope for them just the same;
I'd like to be twenty again;
I'd certainly like to be slim;
I'd also like to be filthy rich,
But living in a nursing home and inflation

Take care of that;
I wish for the world
What men have been wishing for years and years —
I wish for PEACE.
For the country, I would wish we would see
Successful small farmers again;
For the nursing home
I'd wish for lots and lots of nurses,
And when you put the light on,
Someone would come right away,
    or at least in the next twenty minutes;
For my family I'd wish help of some kind —
They shouldn't have to have *all* the responsibility;
And for myself,
I'd certainly wish that I could walk again.

—*Joan Brindley, BRNC*

My wish for the new year
Is for "willingness,"
Willingness to be still
And listen — to wait
And listen for the
Still small voice
To tell me exactly
What to do and say.
"It will come;"
It always does.
The answers always come
And bring such joy,
Whether I like it or not.
Just wait and listen quietly,
"It will come."

—*Dorothy Emerson, BRNC*

PREDICTIONS

So much improvement today
Over what we had when I was a girl —

When I was first married
I had to iron every darn thing!
The future will have lots more things
To make our life easier.
We'll have moving sidewalks
To take us where we want to go—
No more waiting for buses in cold weather!
There will be sightseeing trips on a space shuttle—
Such a trip will not be just for astronauts.
The future will be fascinating—
There will be a cure for cancer.
And best of all,
Someone will come out with a
Nail polish that will stay on.

                                        —Joan Brindley, BRNC

5. The Best Future: Children and Grandchildren

Older people are especially aware of the fact that we live on through our children and grandchildren, and members of my class have always been willing—eager—to write about theirs. A good professional poem is "The Grandson," by James Scully.
   Guidelines:

—Ask how many have children and/or grandchildren and talk for a few minutes about what they like best about them.
—Then ask them to write poems to their children or grandchildren, real or imagined. On the tablet put leading questions: "What are your children or grandchildren like? Describe them, perhaps using metaphors—'My grandson is a spinning top. . . . ,' for example. What do you most wish for them? Be specific. You may wish to talk to them directly in your poem—'Dear _____' and tell them of your hopes."

   Examples:

SIMPLE INNOCENCE

How sweet the innocent child's face is. Clear, and full of hope and truth like a mirror. Be careful and do not mar it with fingerprints and scratches, as discrimination and lost loyalty will mar the

child's face. For something so good and pure should not be lost by
those and other things.

— Stephanie Russek, Grade 6

A grandchild is a new leaf
On the family tree;
We watch closely for traits
That resemble older members —
If the traits are good ones
We encourage them;
If the traits are undesirable
We try to correct them.
Often we correct our own traits
While trying to perfect the child.
The process is mutually beneficial
And brings the generations closer.

— Dorothy Yates, BRNC

Where am I in my granddaughter,
Not too long ago acquired
And living not so near
That I may watch her lovely growth?
Now she toddles,
And in her ever-searching actions
I seek for telltale signs
That mark her as my own;
Her huge eyes and dimpled buttocks
Coyly copy from her mother,
And her father's wide smile and dark curls
Mark her as his;
I am no more important than the silver balloon
Hoisted high on a string
Which suddenly loosens from those small fingers
And lofts just beyond her stretching reach;
She struggles and twists,
Extends her small body and lengthens her grasp,
And grabs the cord and brings back her

Almost lost toy—
And then I know that she is mine.

—*Helen L. Anderson, BRNC*

REFLECTION

Fresh from the floating swans
You feather your sturdy body
With a ragged, homemade tutu,
Bind your spiky hair
In wrinkled silk,
And lock yourself in your room.
Before the mirror
Arms pump,
Plump legs jerk,
Thump
To vibrant Ormandy;
Yet in your shining spring
You see a miracle:
Grace smiles back,
You are one with
Moving beauty.
Daughter, as you grow,
Fall,
Fail,
When soft stabs
Circle you
And you feel like
Brittle ice
Melting among diamonds,
Reach back deep,
Feed on that
Fluid joy.

—*Carol F. Peck*

F. SPECIAL OCCASIONS AND OTHER SPECIFICS

A poem should be
Something that is memorable
And that I can recite
To myself.

—Catherine J. Curtin, BRNC

As most teachers point out, special events, such as holidays, historic occasions, birthdays, etc. provide natural topics for writing, as do objects that can be brought in, passed around, and experienced directly. Other specifics include things in the newspaper—or in the teacher's personal experience—that spark the imagination and lead to a good writing idea.

1. The Yearly Cycle

We all have written poems about seasons, months, holidays—indeed, those turned up in conjunction with other writing ideas in this book. However, working with basically the same people year after year, I have had to go beyond the five senses project, metaphor, form, and memories of the past to find new approaches to the same old topics, to offer new insights into the familiar. Here are a few of the most successful ones:

JANUARY—talk about the Roman god Janus who had two faces, looking backward and forward at the same time—*World Book Encyclopedia* is a good resource; the poem idea is January Visions—what we see when we look backward and when we look forward.

JANUARY VISIONS

Looking back I see Poland in a big turmoil;
Looking ahead I find the U.S.A. and Russia trying to stop the
    arms race.
Looking back I see my grandchildren as babies;
Looking ahead I see them achieving their goals in life.
Looking back I see the Civil War;
Looking ahead I see the races understanding each other.

Looking back I see Nazism in Germany;
Looking ahead I see a strong state of Israel.

—Anna Goldschmidt, BRNC

Looking back I see
All the mountains I did not climb,
All the friends I did not greet,
All the kind deeds I did not do.
Looking ahead
I see another chance—
I plan to do all the things
I have left undone
And to do the good.

—Dorothy Yates, BRNC

FEBRUARY—the idea is "Gloomy February, Magic Me!" Write
about what magic you would like to do to remove the gloom of
February.

GLOOMY FEBRUARY, MAGIC ME!

On a gloomy February day
I would go outside and
With my magic wand
I would change the snow
Into a sun.
Then it would be a
Summer day.

—Charles Leitzell, Kindergarten

In gloomy February
There would definitely be no snow—
I would not allow it;
Buds on the trees would pop,
Flowers would bloom,
Birds would sing;
There would be no wind or rain;

Things that had dormant lain
Would suddenly sprout up;
February would be the best of the year—
The only thing wrong with all this
Is that the lawn would have to be cut!

—Joan Brindley, BRNC

In gloomy February
I would tear the entire page from the calendar;
What would I replace it with?
A gathering of friends exchanging love, warming thoughts
That would expunge the chill and gloom.

—Judith Weinman, BRNC

MARCH—Read Robert Louis Stevenson's poem "The Wind," Christina Rossetti's "Who Has Seen the Wind?" and perhaps Shelley's "Ode to the West Wind;" ask students to talk directly to the March wind and tell it what they like and what they don't like about it.

MARCH WIND

Oh wind, oh wind, where are you going?
Don't you like us here? Because you try to pass away;
Bring us the storm in July,
The snow in December,
Play with the trees, taking down their leaves and ripe apples;
Tell the winter when it should go away;
Bring us spring—everybody yearns for that;
Be mild at the beginning of spring,
But do not blow the blooms off my apple tree too soon;
Wind, oh wind, I love you when you blow my hair,
I love you when you kiss my face,
I love you when you tell me that spring is here;
But I hate you when you blow my airplane around,
When you bring summer storms with dangerous lightning,
And maybe that causes a big fire in California.

—Anna Goldschmidt, BRNC

APRIL — read Chaucer's Prologue to "The Canterbury Tales," Robert Browning's "Home Thoughts From Abroad" and the first part of T. S. Eliot's "Wasteland." Write about "April Dreams," "April Longings," or "April, Cruel or Kind" accordingly.

APRIL DREAMS

The first feeble steps of spring,
Venturing forth, then falling back,
Growing stronger with each attempt,
Promise delicate flowers,
Joyous songs of birds,
Busy humming bees;
A long winter dream of beauty
Becomes reality at last.

— Dorothy Yates, BRNC

APRIL LONGINGS

In April I could leave the city,
Take the only means of transportation, the streetcar,
And spend weekends down on the farm.
The smells were tantalizing —
Skunk cabbage was coming up,
The pine trees were pouring down pine needles
To heap up walls of homes;
School was forgotten.
I was alone,
Imagining,
Planning my future,
A future with Aprils
And dreaming.
How else could I live?

— Dorothy Emerson, BRNC

I long to go to places I haven't been before;
First, every place in the U.S. —
I'd like to go west and see different crops,
    trees and flowers and the people,

To see if they do differently than we do;
I would like to go to England
Because that's where we have gotten most things
And what we have read about;
And I long to pick flowers and look forward
To cutting the hay in hot summer.

—Alice Caton, BRNC

APRIL—CRUEL OR KIND?

April is a month of change—
Out of winter's unrelenting cold
Comes a day of warm sun;
Birds sing, buds appear;
The earth seems bright and happy;
Life is beginning again.
Out of nowhere comes
A sharp, cold wind—
Dark clouds scatter snowflakes;
All life shrinks into itself
To wait for a more hospitable day
When nature bursts forth again
In a joyful song of spring.

—Dorothy Yates, BRNC

MAY—Instead of focusing on usual May celebrations, concentrate on a usually unsung early May flower, the dandelion. The name comes from Old French *dent-de-lion*, or "lion's tooth," (because of the sharply indented leaves), which may suggest a metaphor to somebody. Everybody has *some* association with this flower, and the group enjoyed seeing real dandelions on the table; if you can find some that have gone to seed as well as some in full bloom, you will stir even more memories. Ask the students what it means to them; what their childhood experiences with dandelions were; what it might be a metaphor for, in terms of hardiness, color, and universality; what it looks like to their "new eyes." I called this exercise "One Person's Weed Is Another's Wine."

DANDELIONS

Dandelions mean spring to me.
Then I think of my mother —
She loved them to eat.
We didn't have so many fresh vegetables ninety years ago.
I call them smiles of spring.
Do they grow in Alaska, I wonder?
What is commonplace to us
May be a rarity in other parts of the world.
I never think of them as a common weed
But as the breath of spring,
And smile its welcoming with them.

— Dorothy Emerson, BRNC

What a wonderful subject, the good old dandelion, reliable in forecasting summer, like the robin forecasts spring. Not just one — thousands popping up everywhere there is a grain of dirt, reminding me of my aunts and a certain neighbor who picked the dandelion greens for food and the blossoms for wine. A farm with well-fertilized soil produced thousands of them, and you could see many people in the fields. Yellow, like butter, then turning grey, when the children would pick them to blow the grey away or curl the stems by splitting. I could never reconcile myself to the people in my office who spent their weekends digging up dandelions from their lawns so they would not grow greyheaded and reproduce. The children must have missed the fun.

— Eleanor O'Brien, BRNC

My reaction to dandelions?
I like the dandelion —
It can make the wine
And that can make you feel fine!

— Catherine J. Curtin, BRNC

JUNE — Focus on "June Stories and Glories" — what June means to each writer individually, in terms of personal experiences.

STORIES OF JUNE

June always opened the door to camping—
School was over, but a new education was beginning;
From early years on, I spent summers away from home, in camp;
This meant living in the out-of-doors all summer,
Living with many people my own age,
Learning new crafts, becoming acquainted with nature's world.
Perhaps that is where I learned to meditate—to talk with God.
Until a year or so ago I spent summers teaching 4H Club
    members
What schools never have time to teach.

                                —Dorothy Emerson, BRNC

JUNE CINQUAIN

June
Summer's song
Beckons, ripens, burgeons
Introduced me to earth
Joy

                                 —Carol F. Peck

June
Summer weather
Graduates, brides, and grooms
Finishing or beginning a new life or program.
June 30 used to be
The end of the fiscal year.

                            —Eleanor O'Brien, BRNC

    JULY and *AUGUST*—I have no examples, since I take these months off, but they would lend themselves to the 5 senses treatment, as well as forms like recipes and cinquains.

    SEPTEMBER—For this month my projects have ranged from acrostic poems describing the month (see Chapter C) to less structured poems about what the month awakens in people to a focus on school, which people of this generation seem especially to relate to.

SEPTEMBER AWAKENINGS

September has so many memories —
As the weather got cooler,
Out would come sweaters from the closet;
Sometimes if you waved them right,
You'd get a whiff of mothballs.
Does that wool coat still fit?
The hem will probably have to come up —
They're wearing the clothes shorter this year;
Something else about September:
As soon as everything is out,
The weather will turn warm!

—Joan Brindley, BRNC

CELEBRATE SEPTEMBER

I celebrate September when I see the goldenrod is yellow,
With the childhood poem repeating in my head:
  When the goldenrod is yellow
  And the corn is turning brown,
  And the trees in apple orchard
  With fruit are bending down . . .
And most of all September reminds me of
My freedom by being allowed to go to school
And into the strange unknown outside world
Where you did not take naps and stay home all the time;
Sounds of September were the threshing machine
Which converted the cornstalks from the field into ensilage,
Chopped-up food placed in a high silo
To be fed to the cattle during the winter;
In those days there were not many motorized engines,
Which were in their infancy,
Like the Model T and A Fords.

—Eleanor O'Brien, BRNC

SCHOOL DAYS

Ah, school days —
They seem so long ago!

There were pleasant things
And unpleasant things.
One pleasant thing
Was simply going to school,
Possibly because I was a good student.
An unpleasant thing was that nasty
Little boy in back of me —
His favorite sport seemed to be
Dipping my long hair in the ink well.
Another unpleasant things was trying to
Sit still on those hard wooden seats.
I supposed everyone had a
Favorite and unfavorite subject —
I loved math — later called Algebra and Trigonometry —
I liked them all,
But I sure did hate Chemistry —
I had a teacher who scared me to death.
I imagine whether you did well or not
Depended a lot on the teacher you had;
Let's face it — some people just shouldn't have been teachers.
I wonder if these same teachers made good wives or mothers?

—Joan Brindley, BRNC

OCTOBER — Write a poem welcoming October — and tell it *why* you welcome it.

WELCOME OCTOBER

I like to see October come
Because it changes the menu —
Mincemeat and gingerbread are a relief
From apple pie and cheese,
And Mother always started making coffeekuchen
(It has a lot of raisins in it, and I *love* raisins!).
October always started me off with
Something I didn't like to do — study;
I preferred to play the piano;
I had a Steinway baby grand.
So goodbye to the eats

And hello to hard work!
And goodbye to those days which seemed so bad
But now I see were very good for me!

—Laura Bonesteel, BRNC

I don't know whether to welcome October or not—
I'll be a year older;
How could my mother do that to me,
Have my birthday the same month
As all the other nuts?
On the other hand, in October you see a lot of
My favorite color, yellow;
You see a lot of colors—red, crimson.
Some green is left, but it might be
A different color tomorrow;
Many animals use October for preparing for winter—
Watch the squirrels scurrying around collecting nuts;
The birds are already wondering who is going to feed them
When the ground is covered with a soft blanket of snow;
October is full of smells—
The crisp, clean air of autumn, apples baking,
A stein of beer waiting to disappear;
But here comes a sunny day and warmth
The very day you put all your summer clothing away;
This may be the beginning of winter,
But who's to say?

—Joan Brindley, BRNC

NOVEMBER—Thanksgiving is an expected poetry topic, but
e.e. cummings' poem "i thank You God for most this amazing"
provides an unexpected approach. The unusual word order in the
poem may sound strange to some ears, and I advise reading the
poem aloud at least twice. The writing idea is to use cummings'
first line for poems of general thanksgiving for specific things. Poems about the holiday seem to work best if they pinpoint a specific
Thanksgiving memory.

POEM OF THANKSGIVING

I thank you, God, most for
The love given to me by a nice family;
For the sun shining every nice day,
Making us feel warm and comfortable,
Bringing forth ripening fruits to nourish man and beast;
For health and the feeling of happiness I can enjoy;
For good people living and willing to help others;
For flowers, trees, and all the beauty of nature;
For enjoying a good sleep at night
And waking up refreshed in the morning.

—Anna Goldschmidt, BRNC

I thank you, God,
For colorful stylish clothes
And cooking
And the Bible to read.

—Betty Graham, BRNC

THANKSGIVING MEMORIES

A Thanksgiving in my fairly early childhood I shall never forget, although details are both vague and confused. At our church service program, I can clearly see myself wearing my frilliest pinafore, standing on a table and reciting a poem. Its opening lines were:

I've had my turkey dinner
And don't I look as if I had,
With cranberry sauce and pumpkin pie,
And oh, I am so glad!

There must have followed an enumeration of things I was thankful for, because the final lines were,

But oh! I'm thankfulest of all
Because I didn't have the mumps.

A later Thanksgiving I remember is from our son's early teenage, the period when it is impossible to satisfy their (teenagers') hunger. We were having another family as guests at a traditional Thanksgiving feast, the aromas of which had filled the house since dawn. Our son, Jack, came and said that he was going out for a little while but would be right back. On return, he told us that he'd just gone down to the People's Drug Store at the corner for a sandwich to whet his appetite. Facing an enormous dinner had not deterred him from his trip.

— Vida Hickerson, BRNC

I don't have a memory of a particular Thanksgiving, but one year one of my brothers, in playing cards, won a 23-pound turkey. It was live, so he put it in the basement, which was not finished but still had the dirt floor. The big bread box was kept on a ledge halfway down the stairs. So the family joke was when my mother sent me to get bread. I immediately confronted the big turkey, the first turkey I ever saw, and I never forgot. I did not screech, when I saw him, but ran back up the stairs to the security of the first floor! Needless to say, that year my family had a real Thanksgiving, with all the trimmings, and enough turkey for each one.

—Eleanor O'Brien, BRNC

*DECEMBER—*As with Thanksgiving, holiday poems are best when given a specific focus, such as celebrating gifts: what are the best gifts to give and to receive?

CELEBRATE GIFTS

I'd like to give peace and tranquility to this world—
If you have peace you have everything;
Then people could be with their children.
My favorite gifts to receive:
Flowers blooming outside—I never get enough of that—
Snowy days,
And all music!

—Pauline Immerman, BRNC

To give makes one glow
With the warm feeling of
Generosity, friendship and thought;

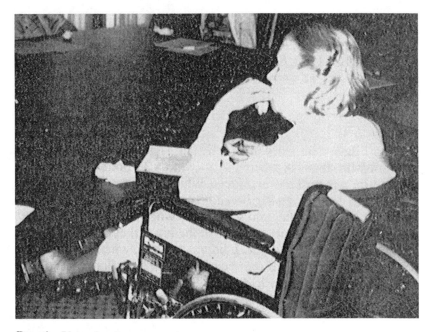

Dorothy Yates has been an active member of the class since its first meeting in 1978.

Photo by Wendy C. Webster.

We give part of ourselves
And receive back a flood of love;
Little stars of understanding
Pass between giver and receiver
And light the universe of humanity.

—Dorothy Yates, BRNC

The greatest gift that can be given is free to give
And longingly sought by everyone;
We beg for it in everything we do,
No matter what our art.
The genius is not without it
And the idiot becomes renewed by its extension.
The child must learn to use it

While feasting on its produce.
The old already have so much
And often do not use it well.
The gift is best when equally shared,
And no gift at all can equal
That wonderful trade of human understanding!

—Helen Anderson, BRNC

I was describing myself as being in my late 90's,
But I discovered that actually I am in my late 80's,
So a great gift is the gift of accuracy!
If you hit your age wrong
It will put the children off
And everything!

—John Mann, BRNC

2. Terrific Tangibles

All writing teachers know that tangible objects can really spark imaginations and memories. Students love the surprise of something they can experience with all five senses firsthand. Whatever I bring in, I try to have enough that each person can have his or her own to touch, smell, taste and look at, especially people with limited vision. Once in a while someone who has not understood the lesson, or who seldom writes, will come to life when handed a flower or fruit. The writing projects still need some focus and direction, however. Some tangibles I have had success with are:

DAFFODILS—These are a natural for spring writing and touch off many memories; occasionally I have read Wordsworth's "The Daffodils," suggested talking to them, or suggested a metaphoric approach—are they spring's old-fashioned telephones?

ON DAFFODILS

You look lovely,
You feel beautiful,
You smell like summer is around the corner!
I think you are beautiful

And you make me feel great.
Be a good girl and behave yourself!

—Pauline Immerman, BRNC

Bright yellow trumpets
Sounding the welcome arrival of spring,
They bring cheer and hope
To winter-weary earth;
They promise more beauty to come
And make us happy to be alive
In an awakening world.

—Dorothy Yates, BRNC

Daffodils—I think of young girls dressed in yellow,
Their petticoats dancing in the breeze;
I love their smell—it reminds me of spring;
Their petals feel crinkly;
They are a celebration of spring!

—Catherine J. Curtin, BRNC

PANSIES—I told the class where the name came from (French *pensees*, meaning "thoughts,") and asked them to write down the thoughts stirred in them by the flowers.

PANSY THOUGHTS

Pansies do not always wait for spring,
But early in the year make hearts sing
With their little monkey faces
Peeping from unexpected places;
Some have brown eyes, others blue,
Making so many colors of such rich hues;
We look for them to use again,
To press in books and put in frames,
And have you ever heard of a nicer name?

—Marie Huff, BRNC

Colorful little faces
Peering up from the ground,
Each a different color, a different mood;
Some are happy, some sad,
All are new to the world;
Each in its brief life span
Is seeking the meaning of creation,
Bringing beauty and wonder to the earth.

—Dorothy Yates, BRNC

MARIGOLDS—Students liked the origin of the name, "Mary's gold," and the fact that it is a native of Mexico, and I suggested that they talk to the flower, listen to what it was saying, or use a metaphoric approach. The marigolds I brought in were the two-tone, French variety.

ON MARIGOLDS

It is beautiful and has its own individuality—
One stem has several possibilities;
It is so unusual you are speechless;
Mine has a tiny inchworm measuring it,
But that's the shortest inch I've ever seen—
Do they always grow to fit the flower?

—Elizabeth Hood, BRNC

Marigolds—I think they are beautiful;
I used to have so many
I didn't know what to do with them;
Mine has a worm, too—
I'd say to him, "Get out of my flower!"

—John Mann, BRNC

Obviously the name—marry gold—means marry money;
As I look at it further, other things come to mind:
The yellow (or gold) center reminds me of the Aztec calendar;
I know better than to explore it with my nose;

I touch the flower I have,
And the dark outside petals have the feel of velvet;
What does it say to me?
It says: "I'll be around long after other things have gone."

—Joan Brindley, BRNC

Marigolds are like the Washington Redskins—
Their colors are burgundy and gold;
They have a single root system
And branch up and out in shaggy greenery;
Some bloom bigger and more successfully than others,
    who don't quite make it,
Just like incompleted forward passes;
The biggest and brightest are the Hogs—
They have a useful purpose,
And even though they seem tough and masculine,
They can be surprisingly fragile;
In fact, life is like that, too.

—Dorothy Ahrens, BRNC

TOMATOES (when my garden overflowed)—these almost demanded the five-senses approach which led naturally to memories.

TOMATO CELEBRATIONS

A tomato is sort of the
Harbinger of fall colors:
First green,
Then yellow,
Then finally red.
How the birds love its seeds!
How we love tomatoes,
Sometimes in a salad,
Sometimes stewed,
Sometimes "as is."

—Joan Brindley, BRNC

A glowing red ball
That draws its color and
Glows from the sun;
As the sun warms the earth
The tomato warms the palate,
Making the senses grow stronger
As the plant grows taller,
Ending in a glowing red ball of
Pleasure and beauty.

—Dorothy Yates, BRNC

MILKWEED—I brought in both green pods and a jar full of the
ripe seeds. After reading Richard Wilbur's "Two Voices in a
Meadow: A Milkweed and A Stone" and some children's metaphors, I asked them to look at the milkweed with their own "new
eyes" and write metaphors.

MILKWEED METAPHORS

Milkweed pods are . . .
A prickly green claw,
Two green mustaches.
A milkweed seed is . . .
A spaceship for a small Martian.

—Paul More, Grade 2

Milkweed pods are . . .
Two bees' bodies sitting by each other,
Two fingernails of a giant witch.
A milkweed seed is a fan.

—Mikol Rudd, Grade 2

NEW EYES ON MILKWEED

Looking at these two green things stuck together
Like two beans on a stalk, one never would guess
What miracles they have inside.
Inside they have witches' brooms,

Thin white hair on a brown handle,
Dandelion seeds on a stick,
White cotton growing out of a brown body,
A fairy strewing goods around,
A doll with silvery hair, very beautiful,
Snow White sitting on a brown chair,
A parachute dropping out of an airplane.

—Anna Goldschmidt, BRNC

A rough, forbidding pod
Holds its inner secrets
Safe from inquiring eyes;
Gradually the warmth of the sun
Opens the reluctant doors
And small fairy fountains
Fly swiftly into the
Waiting world.

—Dorothy Yates, BRNC

AMARYLLIS—In January, when little else was blooming, this commanded attention and awe and begged to be spoken or listened to—I did not need one for each member! I suggested a 3-line approach, synthesizing the experience.

AMARYLLIS

The stamens speak to me,
Although surrounded by a silken cup of rose,
They sing their siren song.

—Helen Day, BRNC

First a long green bud,
Then an explosion of color
So sudden as to be mystical.

—Helen Day, BRNC

A cornucopia of beauty —
Rich shimmering red,
A world of happiness held within.

—Dorothy Yates, BRNC

It takes me to church
Where I hear silence
Soft and red.

—Betty Graham, BRNC

3. Tributes

Occasionally the poets have written tributes to various people or things, such as their nurses, special friends, and even the human hand, showing their appreciation through specifics. (See the group tribute to their nurses in Section 3.)

TRIBUTE TO THE NURSES

A lady named Nightingale
Opened her heart to those in need
Until the need was lovingly met —
Pain was eliminated
And replaced with comfort and smiles;
Despair was replaced by hope.

—Judith Weinman, BRNC

The nurses are very good to me;
I like having them around me;
I like to talk and joke with them —
They are kind and loving —
They are my family!

—Sarah McInteer, BRNC

Nurses come in all sizes and shapes
And can give a pill or patch one with tape;
They let us know they are always near
To soothe a pain or calm a fear;

They are here both night and day
With a cheery word to say;
Now we can say a sincere thank you
for all the many things you do.

—Marie Huff, BRNC

FRIENDS

Friends are a rock
Upon whom the storms of our lives beat;
They break the adverse forces
Rushing toward us;
They bring safety and comfort
To our battered lives,
A haven of peace and comfort
Enduring always.

—Dorothy Yates, BRNC

A special friend of mine passed away recently;
I shall always miss her—
She used to give me a call by phone every week;
She was as reliable as the day
Coming back after the night;
I shall never forget all the goodness
I got from her;
When she died, her daughter said:
"Only angels die that way."
I replied, "Don't you know that she was an angel?"

—Anna Goldschmidt, BRNC

A friend is one you can't get along without;
She shows this all the time,
Because she is such a good friend.
You can depend on her—
She's never missing when you want her.
She is like a really good book—
Always there with the right words,
Dependable,

But you couldn't buy her,
You could never pay for her.
She is dependable in a way
You couldn't expect in a piece of paper!

—*Dorothy Oest, BRNC*

HANDS, WOW!

Hands can play volleyball with the greatest of ease,
But feet cannot;
Hands can pick flowers, oh, so easily,
As feet break them in half;
Hands can play and write a letter today;
Hands can welcome people to your house;
Hands can read Braille, wow!

—*Julia Davis, Grade 3*

The hands of man are an extension of his soul
And ever a servant to his devouring eyes;
Hands have no gift to give or life to live—
Whatever they proffer with tapered beauty,
Dimpled innocence or age-clawed form,
It is offered from another source;
Hands make love, great paintings,
And music to shred the soul;
Hands build walls and castles,
And shining spans,
And dishes and iron pots;
And hands make war
And undo much they have done;
And hands can talk,
But it's always the mind that plots the action
And reaps benefits on which to thrive.

—*Helen L. Anderson, BRNC*

A human hand can do many, many things—
It helps to change the diaper
On the new baby;

The hand points toward heaven
As the young child kneels by her bed,
Waiting to leap between the sheets;
All its life it puts food into our mouths;
It waves goodbye at the train station or airport;
It wears the wedding ring
That announces to the world
This person belongs to somebody;
A hand sometimes has the opportunity of
Saving a life in the operating room;
And what scratches your nose when it itches?
A hand.

—Joan Brindley, BRNC

4. The Ultimate Special Occasion

National Nursing Home Week occurs in May, and several times I was able to take a group of six or eight fourth graders over to join the group and write with them on that year's theme, such as "Love Is Ageless," "Memories Are Made To Be Shared," and "Celebrate Life's Achievements." I interspersed the children among the elderly and gave everyone a chance to get acquainted. I was never prouder of both groups, and best of all, everyone relaxed and had a good time — before and after giving serious attention to their writing, of course. After writing, all the poets read their work out loud and were mutually appreciative.

A WELCOME POEM TO OUR 4TH GRADE VISITORS

Oh wonderful creatures
    still ungrown,
Your first decade
Loosely spread
    behind you,
What unused magic
    is readying
The not yet measured
    height of you?

But your greatest size
   will never be enough
To guard the gloried
   talents your small
Frames forever nourish
To be slowly swirled
   into the fullness
   of us all.

                     —Helen L. Anderson, BRNC

MEMORIES

The big house on the hill
That we often visited
Has become a museum now;
When I was little
I went down the hill
To see a little boy
I was not supposed to see
Because he was a "bad example" —
But I just loved him.
Since I am grown I realize that
He must have had something in him
And I in me that made me love him,
Because he grew up to become a preacher
In a small town in Iowa.
So up hill or down dale,
We never know how character grows.

                     —Laura Bonesteel, BRNC

I had a blanket
That I slept with
   and wept with;
Sitting here thinking
   brings back some
Memories I never knew I had
   and now they are
   in my head like

The pencil is in my hand,
Thoughts of sliding
  and thoughts of
riding,
      thinking of
playing in the
         rain
when I was five,
  thinking of sledding
   in the snow
  when I was six;
  Funny how thoughts
      of a little
       blanket
  can remind me of
singing and playing in my head
   like a rubber
   ball bouncing
   back and forth,
        up and down.

                — *V.W. Fowlkes, Grade 4*

As the years accumulate
Our most vivid memories are of the past;
The people who most influenced our lives
Loom large and we see how
They guided our thoughts and interests.
A neighbor took me on bird walks,
Another neighbor helped me to identify wild flowers,
A high school teacher gave me an abiding interest in literature,
Another in history,
And all through our growing period
Our parents directed our health, our minds
  and our spiritual lives;
Today we are the product of our memories.

                — *Dorothy Yates, BRNC*

CELEBRATE LIFE'S ACHIEVEMENTS

What I thought was a nice little hobby years ago
Turned out to be quite different —
I began to collect seashells in the Virgin Islands
(All old people collect something);
I displayed them,
Lectured about them,
And in a way, I was famous.
By this time, the collection numbered
In the thousands.
One day something came along,
Mowed me down, and put me in a wheel chair;
I wasn't very old at the time, but
Accidents don't ask your age.
Today my name is on a plaque in the Virgin Islands —
One door announces "The Joan S. Brindley Collection" —
You'd think I really was somebody —
I couldn't be more surprised!
And to prove I didn't dream all this,
My family has pictures of this.

—*Joan Brindley, BRNC*

In my first year of my life it was walking, crawling, and saying
  some sounds;
In the second year of my life I started talking and running like the
  wind (and I got into the terrible two's);
In the third year of my life I started jumping, talking in complete
  sentences, and, most of all, sharing;
In the fourth year of my life I went to school and learned how to
  write the alphabet down;
In the fifth year of my life I learned how to read basic books and
  write some words;
In the sixth year of my life I learned how to read and write more;
In the seventh year of my life I learned by myself how to ride a
  bicycle!
In the eighth year of my life I did a play called "No Talking"
  and I got shot in it;

In the ninth year of my life I did a play called "The Twins On
    Vernacular Island" and I was a leading role;
We've gone through all of my life's achievements;
Now I am in the tenth year of my life, and every day I achieve
    something.

— Trevor Boerger, Grade 4

5. Potpourri — Look Around You

I used to worry that I would run out of topics for the group to
write about, but I have discovered that life abounds with ideas, if
you are receptive. The daily newspaper often has articles that spark
ideas, such as the essay on September awakenings, filled with vivid
imagery, that I used as an example one year. When my daughter
gave her senior piano recital, I took in the tape and played the first
two numbers, familiar Bach pieces, and asked the group to describe
what the music made them think of and how it made them feel.
When the same daughter was planning her wedding and receiving a
great deal of advice from many sources, I read Polonius' advice to
Laertes (*Hamlet*, Act I, Scene iii) to the poets and asked them to
write the "advice" poems. And it was my mother's mention of her
secret desire to be a jockey and ride the Kentucky Derby winner that
sparked the "secret desire" projects. After an educational trip
around the British Isles, I showed my slides to the group, one edited
box per session — not as just passive viewing, which abounds in
nursing homes, but as an activity — they knew they would have to
connect with the slides through writing. I asked them to describe
what it would be like to live in a castle, what they thought the
various stone circles, such as Stonehenge and the Ring of Brodgar,
signified, what wonders and emotions the cathedrals stirred in
them, what it would be like to live in a Stone Age village like Skara
Brae, and what it would be like to be royalty for a day.

Other special events that generated ideas were Earth Day, for
which we wrote poems *to* the earth, telling it what we loved about it
and asking it to teach us some of its qualities, and the reappearance
of Halley's Comet in March, 1986 — the second time around for
most of the poets; we considered the idea of riding on a comet and
what we might see and feel. One of the most popular special days

was the collective birthday—I had discovered that three of our members had May birthdays, one of which fell on a workshop day, so I baked cupcakes, put a small candle in each, and we sang to each other and wrote about "A Memorable Birthday." We even wrote about "Shoes," an idea stemming from my sorting out several pairs and thinking about the various shoes one wears in a lifetime.

Some of the ideas have come from the residents themselves. When writing on another topic, a member mentioned the A. E. Housman poem, "When I Was One and Twenty," so the next week we all wrote about being twenty-one—what was going on in the world, what was going on in our lives, whether or not we would like to be twenty-one again, and why, and whether or not we would do anything differently if we had another chance. And one lady, Joan Brindley, regularly contributed such writing ideas as: "What things in this world do we *not* need, such as mosquitos?" "Professions I would not want"; "Were 'the good old days' really that good?" and "Things you don't see any more," such as corsets and dish towels. Another time we were writing "moon poems," and one lady wrote that all she could think of was "The moon was a ghostly galleon, tossed upon cloudy seas" from Alfred Noyes' "The Highwayman," and there was a pleased murmur of recognition—so next session we had a rousing good time when I read "The Highwayman" aloud apropos of nothing but enjoying a favorite poem together. And I learned not to be so intent on the topic or technique of the moment that I missed a possible connection.

Always I have tried to stay tuned into the collective experiences of the group. You never know what memory you will tap into, or when it will happen. What matters is that when it does happen, you delight in it—for example, when we were doing April poems and I happened to read Chaucer's "Prologue" to *The Canterbury Tales*, one lady who up to then had not been very responsive suddenly joined me, quoting flawlessly in Middle English, and suddenly felt connected with poetry through her past experience. That made me realize all over again that I was working with intelligent, educated, feeling people with very different personalities and that even though most of my experience was with children, all writing classes share the excitement of words and ideas—and the nursing home group had the advantage of drawing on lifetimes of experience, rather than pretending.

POETRY CLASS

I had a terrible headache
But I came to Poetry Group anyway,
And I heard the thoughts of others
Who had really experienced life —
A medical student's or
A theologian's advice
Would not have done me as much good
As hearing from the lips of those who had lived —
It was better than any pill!

—*Laura Bonesteel, BRNC*

Afterword

I now know what "labor of love" means. As I have gone through ten years' worth of poems, to put this book together, I have been struck all over again by the quality of this writing by people who never before thought of themselves as poets. The truth, the beauty in their work says something about the strength and beauty of the human spirit. Working with their poems I have felt connected with these people, with poetry, with my own life history—with humanity in general and my own private center in particular. I have seen anew what I always knew: connection is all.

Bibliography

ANTHOLOGIES

Some of the following anthologies contain poems for adults; others, as noted, contain poems written for children but good for any age. I include several of those, because the elderly seem especially to enjoy hearing again poems they knew and memorized as children.

Dore, Anita, ed. *The Premier Book of Major Poets*. Greenwich, Conn.: Fawcett Publications, Inc., 1970.

Ellmann, Richard, ed. *The New Oxford Book of American Verse*. New York: Oxford University Press, 1976.

Hubbard, Alice, and Babbitt, Adeline, ed. *The Golden Flute*, An Anthology of Poetry for Young Children. New York: John Day Company, 1932. (This anthology contains an excellent index by topics.)

Larrick, Nancy, ed. *Piping Down the Valleys Wild*, Poetry for the Young of All Ages. New York: Delacorte Press, 1968.

New Yorker Editors. *The New Yorker Book of Poems*. New York: Morrow Quill Paperbacks, 1974.

Smith, A.J.M., ed. *Seven Centuries of Verse, English & American*. New York: Charles Scribner's Sons, 1967.

Sullivan, Nancy, ed. *The Treasury of American Poetry*. Garden City, N.Y.: Doubleday & Company, Inc., 1978.

Untermeyer, Louis, ed. *A Treasury of Great Poems*. New York: Simon and Schuster, 1942.

Untermeyer, Louis, ed. *Rainbow in the Sky*. (For children) New York: Harcourt, Brace & World, Inc., 1935.

Untermeyer, Louis, ed. *The Golden Treasury of Poetry*. (For children) New York: Golden Press, 1959.

ANTHOLOGIES OF WRITING BY CHILDREN

Exley, Richard & Helen, ed. *To Grandma & Grandpa*. Boston: Houghton Mifflin Company, 1979.

Joseph, Stephen M., ed. *the me nobody knows*. New York: Avon Books, 1969.

Lewis, Richard, ed. *Journeys*, Prose by children of the English-speaking world. New York: Simon and Schuster, 1969.

Lewis, Richard, ed. *Miracles*, Poems by children of the English-speaking world. New York: Simon and Schuster, 1966.

IDEA BOOKS

Artists & Elders Backlist — a group of books available from Teachers & Writers Collaborative, 5 Union Square West, New York, N.Y. 10003. (Write for their catalogue.) Books include:

• *The Journal Project*, by Kaminsky
• *Talking Poetry, Hablando Poesia,* by Bloom
• *Lives at Sea*, by Worsley
• *Over the Years*, by Wright
• *Blood, Fire and Pillars of Smoke*, by Green

Coberly, Lenore; McCormick, Jeri; and Updike, Karen. *Writers Have No Age: Creative Writing with Older Adults*. New York: The Haworth Press, 1984.

Cowles, Fleur. *If I Were An Animal*. New York: William Morrow and Company, Inc., 1986.

Heartland Journal, 4114 North Sunset Court, Madison, Wisconsin 53705. "A magazine by writers over 60 for readers of all ages." 3 issues per year.

Koch, Kenneth. *I Never Told Anybody*, Teaching Poetry Writing in a Nursing Home. New York: Vintage Books (A Division of Random House), 1978. (Includes poems by the residents.)

Koch, Kenneth. *Rose, where did you get that red?* Teaching great poetry to children. New York: Vintage Books, 1974. (Includes poems by children.)

Koch, Kenneth. *Wishes, Lies, and Dreams*. New York: Vintage Books, (A Division of Random House), 1970.

O'Neill, Mary. *Hailstones and Halibut Bones*. Garden City, N.Y.: Doubleday & Co., 1961.

Padgett, Ron. *Handbook of Poetic Forms*. New York: Teachers & Writers Collaborative, 1987.

Slung, Michele. *Momilies*. New York: Ballantine Books, 1985.

The Write Age, First Magazine of Writing Therapy. P.O. Box 722, Menomonee Falls, Wisconsin 53051.

Williams, William Carlos. *Selected Poems*. New York: New Directions, 1969.

Willis, Meredith Sue. *Personal Fiction Writing*, A Guide to Writing from Real Life for Teachers, Students, & Writers. New York: Teachers & Writers Collaborative, 1984.

Viorst, Judith. *If I Were In Charge Of The World (and other worries)*. New York: Atheneum, 1981.

REFERENCE BOOKS

Childcraft and *World Book Encyclopedia*. Chicago, Illinois: Field Enterprises Educational Corporation, 1967. (Available in the children's section of any public library.)